DIABETES:
Questions You Have ... Answers You Need

DIABETES:

Questions You Have ... Answers You Need

Paula Brisco

Consultant editor Dr Robert Youngson

Thorsons
An Imprint of HarperCollinsPublishers

Thorsons
An Imprint of HarperCollins*Publishers*
77–85 Fulham Palace Road,
Hammersmith, London W6 8JB
1160 Battery Street,
San Francisco, California 94111–1213

Published by Thorsons 1997
3 5 7 9 10 8 6 4

A catalogue record for this book
is available from the British Library

ISBN 0 7225 3307 1

Printed and bound in Great Britain by
Caledonian International Book Manufacturing Ltd, Glasgow

CONTENTS

PUBLISHER'S NOTE

No popular medical book, however detailed, can ever be considered a substitute for consultation with, or the advice of, a qualified doctor. This is especially so in the case of a popular book on a disease like diabetes. This is a condition that requires continuous and close medical supervision. You will find much in this book that may be of the greatest importance to your health and wellbeing, but the book is not intended to replace your doctor or to discourage you from seeking his or her advice.

If anything in this book leads you to suppose that you may be suffering from any of the diabetic complications with which it is concerned, you are urged to see your doctor immediately. Every effort has been made to ensure that the contents of this book reflect current medical opinion and that it is as up to date as possible, but it does not claim to contain the last word on any medical matter.

Terms printed in **boldface** can be found in the glossary, beginning on *page 170*. Only the first mention of the word in the text is emboldened.

INTRODUCTION

It will hardly be necessary to tell you that diabetes is not a condition to be taken lightly. In spite of remarkable recent advances and real promise of an effective cure at some time in the future, it is still an incurable disease. The one thing that is special about diabetes is that the outcome – essentially, whether or not you (or the young person for whom you are responsible) suffer damaging complications – depends on you. Proper medical care and advice are, of course, essential, but they cannot ensure that the disease is properly managed. Your doctor cannot be with you every day.

There are two aims in the management of diabetes – to avoid complications and to live a normal life, with no restrictions on activity, for a full lifespan. People with normal pancreatic function, whose blood-sugar levels are normally controlled and kept within the acceptable limits, do not develop the complications of diabetes. This may seem self-evident – as obvious as saying that people without diabetes haven't got diabetes. But it is actually an important thought. It implies that people who can achieve the kind of standards of blood-sugar control that the healthy body achieves for itself can avoid diabetic complications.

You are not going to be able to do this unless you know quite a lot about diabetes. It is not enough to have a few general facts about the disease; you must know, and clearly understand, at least as much about it as the average GP. This is a subject about which you must become a real specialist. *Diabetes: Questions You Have ... Answers You Need* will help you to acquire this knowledge and understanding. The book is based on real questions that people with diabetes have asked, so it is very much to the point. Just about every question you could possibly ask is posed in this book, and all of them are answered in detail. You may even find answers to questions you may never have thought of asking.

Diabetes is a serious and potentially dangerous condition, but with this expertise, coupled with qualified medical treatment, there is no reason why you should not live an entirely normal and satisfying life.

Dr R. M. Youngson, Series Editor
London, 1997

CHAPTER ONE

THE BASICS

Q **What is diabetes?**
A Diabetes is a malfunction in the body's ability to convert **carbohydrates** – sweet and starchy foods, such as fruit, bread and vegetables – into energy to power the body. The medical name for this is **diabetes mellitus**, meaning 'honey-sweet diabetes'. As you might gather from such a name, diabetes is characterized by an abnormally high and persistent concentration of sugar in the bloodstream (doctors often refer to this as 'raised blood sugar') and in the urine. From time immemorial the condition has been diagnosed by tasting the urine. Other character-istics, besides sugar in the urine, are excessive urine production and unusual thirst, hunger and weight loss. People affected with diabetes generally require lifelong medical- and self-care to control the disease.

Q **Why are carbohydrates a problem?**
A The problem is not so much the carbohydrates as such, but the way the body uses them to create energy. The process of converting food into energy is called

metabolism, and diabetes is often called a metabolic disorder. To explain why carbohydrates pose a problem, let's look first at the metabolic system of a healthy person.

In a normal body, carbohydrates are converted to glucose and other simple sugars in the small intestine. Glucose moves from the intestine into the veins. The blood circulates glucose through the body, where it goes to the liver, muscle and fat cells, either to be stored for later use or to be used immediately as energy. Thus, glucose enters body cells, powering the muscles, heart and brain and assisting the body in maintaining a constant temperature.

A body of a person with diabetes also converts carbohydrates to sugars and sends them into the blood. But at this point things begin to go wrong: the glucose has trouble getting into the cells.

Q   **Why is that?**
A   The answer has to do with **insulin**, a hormone that enables the body to burn carbohydrates.

Q   **Insulin? Where does that come from?**
A   It comes from the **pancreas** – a 15-cm (6-in) long gland that is located behind the stomach. In healthy people, the pancreas secretes many fluids, including insulin. However, in a person with diabetes, one of two things happens: No insulin – or not enough insulin – is being produced by the pancreas, or what the pancreas does produce is not functioning properly. In either case, the system has gone

awry; the end result is that most of the glucose remains in the blood and cannot be processed as energy.

Q So insulin is important?

A Absolutely. That one hormone enables the cells to absorb glucose for use as energy. Without it, a 'glucose glut' eventually results – high levels of unused sugar are trapped in the bloodstream.

Q How high?

A Blood-glucose levels vary during the course of the day. In normal adults, blood-glucose levels range between 3.5 and 5.6 mmol/L (60 and 100 milligrams per decilitre – designated as mg/dl) of blood plasma when a person is **fasting**. By fasting, the medical profession means that the person hasn't eaten for 3 or more hours (before breakfast, for example). Blood-glucose figures are slightly higher for children.

When fasting blood sugar is between 5.6 and 6.4 mmol/L (115 and 140 mg/dl), doctors become mildly concerned. If your doctor runs multiple fasting tests on your blood and the results are over 7.8 mmol/L (140 mg/dl), you are considered to have diabetes. In short, your blood-sugar levels are too high.

Q So what's wrong with high blood sugar?

A As sugar builds in the bloodstream, the kidneys try to pump it out. To eliminate the sugar, the kidneys must dissolve it. The more sugar there is to be eliminated, the more urine must be passed.

You can see how this situation quickly leads to frequent urination, increased thirst and dehydration – three of the symptoms of diabetes. The kidneys can effectively keep the body from becoming overrun with sugar, but, in many cases, their function eventually breaks down. This is not, as you may think, because they have to work harder, but for another reason that we will come to in due course. At this stage, just bear in mind that uncontrolled diabetes can eventually bring on kidney failure.

But that's not the only problem with high blood sugar.

Q   **What's the other?**

A   At the same time that the kidneys are furiously flushing the system of sugar, the body is seriously low on fuel. The body's cells, unable to burn sugar, begin to use protein and body fat as sources of energy.

This breakdown of fats for fuel releases toxic acids called **ketones**. Some ketones are excreted through the urine. Eventually, however, the ketones accumulate, and at high levels they can lead to a condition called **ketoacidosis**, which is in effect a poisoning of the system. Initial symptoms of this are frequent urination, increased thirst and dry mouth, the latter a result of dehydration. In extreme cases, ketoacidosis can cause unconsciousness – what is known as **diabetic coma**. If left untreated, ketoacidosis can kill.

Q **So you're saying that diabetes can be life-threatening?**

A Definitely. The very nature of the disease puts the sufferer at risk of serious complications. Some experts believe diabetes is now the third or fourth leading cause of death.

Q **What can happen if diabetes goes unchecked?**

A Diabetes hastens wear and tear on many crucial bodily functions. In particular, it attacks:

- the circulatory system, leading to coronary heart disease, stroke and blood supply problems in the hands and feet. These conditions are two to four times more common in people with diabetes, and they account for most of their hospitalizations. Heart attacks, hardening of the arteries, strokes, poor circulation in the feet, amputations – these are concrete and common examples of diabetes damage.
- the kidneys. Diabetes is the leading cause of end-stage kidney disease.
- the eyes. Diabetic eye disease, or diabetic **retinopathy**, is the major cause of new serious loss of vision in people 20 to 74 years old.
- the nervous system. Nerve cells may be disturbed or damaged, causing severe pain or loss of feeling – a condition known as **neuropathy**.

We examine the complications of diabetes in Chapter 4. For now, it suffices to say that diabetes must be treated seriously. In nearly all situations, people with diabetes require, at a minimum, routine medical treatment – including daily self-care.

Left unchecked, diabetes shortens life. It is not a condition that goes away.

Q **What can be done about it?**

A Quite simply, you must learn to control your diabetes – don't let it control you! Many people with diabetes have taken personal responsibility for managing their disease and, as a result, they live normal, productive lives. If any disorder can be called a lifestyle disease, diabetes comes as close as any. Just by controlling blood sugar, the severity of diabetic complications can be prevented.

So, the most obvious step is to get blood-sugar levels down to normal. For some people, this means taking insulin; for others, it means losing weight; for some, it means both. For all people with diabetes, it means paying particular attention to diet and exercise – what we mean by a lifestyle change.

All of the experts in the field recount the importance of sound health habits that can help control diabetes and, in some cases, prevent it. You'll find plenty of hands-on information about managing diabetes in this book, and we'll guide you to additional resources.

But whatever their lifestyles, the very first step for all people with diabetes is to find out that they have the disease and to realize that they are not alone.

Q How many people have diabetes?

A In the world, probably well over 100 million. In Britain, between 600,000 and 1 million people have diabetes. That includes people of all ages, from children to the elderly. And the number is increasing steadily. Perhaps 40 per cent of these people are unaware that they have diabetes.

Q You mean some people have diabetes and don't know it?

A Yes.

Q How can that be?

A Scientists estimate that the onset of the disease can be anywhere from 4 to 12 years prior to the fact becoming obvious. That means someone may have diabetes 5, 8, even 10 years before it is diagnosed, depending upon the kind of diabetes that person has. Unfortunately, in that time the condition can damage the body.

Many people only find out about their diabetes once they start having trouble with their eyes, nerves, kidneys, blood vessels or heart.

Q Is there more than one kind of diabetes?

A Yes. Although people tend to think of diabetes as one disease, it is really a group of disorders. What they all have in common is a problem with insulin production or insulin action.

Q   Can you give some examples of the different disorders?

A   Let's start by looking at the two most common, **type-I diabetes** and **type-II diabetes**.

TYPE-1 DIABETES

Q   What is this?

A   Type-I diabetes is the most severe form of diabetes. It is also known as **insulin-dependent diabetes**. People with type-I diabetes depend on injections of insulin to regulate their sugar metabolism. In the past, type-I diabetes was called **juvenile diabetes** because doctors thought it would strike only children or young adults. Doctors now know that people of any age can develop type-I diabetes, although the majority of cases are discovered in people under 20 years of age.

People with type-I diabetes are vulnerable to dangerous short-term complications of the disease. Two of these complications have to do with disruptive swings in blood-sugar levels, such as **hyperglycaemia** (too much blood sugar) and **hypoglycaemia** (too little blood sugar). People with type-I diabetes are also at particular risk of ketoacidosis – that dangerous build-up of toxic acids in the body mentioned earlier.

Q   How many people have type-I diabetes?

A   Almost all Caucasian children with diabetes have type-I, while about 10 per cent of adults with diabetes have type-I. But even that fraction translates into a very large number.

Q **What causes it?**

A Experts call type-I diabetes an **autoimmune** disease and suggest that it is genetically programmed. (*Autoimmune* is a term used to describe what happens when the body's immune system attacks itself.) Here is what happens:

Inside the pancreas are approximately 100,000 cell clusters known as the **islets of Langerhans**, or **islets**. Each islet may include 1,000 to 2,000 **beta cells**, which manufacture insulin and release it into the bloodstream when blood-glucose levels rise. These cells actually monitor the levels of blood sugar and respond to a rise by automatically producing more insulin. In people with type-I diabetes, beta cells are attacked by the immune system and are slowly destroyed. Eventually the production of insulin comes to a halt because no beta cells remain.

Scientists are not quite sure what causes the body's immune system to sabotage these pancreatic cells, although they have detected a genetic predisposition to this disorder. Many scientists also believe that a trigger, perhaps a virus infection, must be present to start the destruction. This theory is supported by the fact that a few cases of type-I diabetes, caught at this early stage, have actually been cured by means of **immunosuppressive drugs**. By blocking the self-destructive action of the immune system, the damage to the islet cells has been checked and full health restored.

Q **How long does this destruction take?**

A Probably 4 to 7 years, according to recent research. Unfortunately, symptoms don't arise until 80 to 90 per cent of the beta cells have been destroyed. Once that happens, sudden and dramatic symptoms appear. The disease is easily detected and quickly diagnosed at that point.

Q **What are the symptoms?**

A They include frequent urination, constant thirst and hunger, and rapid weight loss. Some people suffer from fatigue, blurred vision and recurrent skin infections. Medical tests show sugar in the urine and elevated blood-sugar levels.

TYPE-II DIABETES

Q **What is meant by type-II?**

A Type-II is often called **non-insulin-dependent diabetes**. Formerly called **adult-onset diabetes** or **maturity-onset diabetes**, it seldom develops in people under the age of 40. However, experts are quick to point out that age is an unreliable indicator of diabetes type, since a person of any age can develop type-II diabetes. Type-II diabetes in children and adolescents, affecting some 5 per cent of young people with diabetes, is sometimes called **maturity-onset diabetes of the young** and given the acronym MODY. Some of these diabetes sufferers have a strong family history of the disease.

Q   **How common is type-II diabetes?**

A   It accounts for some 85 to 90 per cent of all cases of diabetes, and usually shows up in middle-aged to older adults. Four out of five of these people are overweight – and in most cases, these people were overweight *before* their diabetes developed.

To an even greater extent than with type-I, type-II runs in families. But it's generally thought that a combination of excess weight and age triggers the existing genetic predisposition.

Q   **How else does type-I diabetes differ from type-II?**

A   A major difference is that people with type-I diabetes must use insulin to live. Their bodies cannot produce this hormone because their beta cells have been irrevocably destroyed. Although some people with type-II diabetes eventually become insulin dependent, most can produce enough insulin to control their sugar levels through some combination of drugs, weight loss, diet and exercise.

The biggest difference is that people with type-II diabetes, by controlling their disease, are able to reverse the disease process so that the insulin produced is adequate to achieve normal function.

Q   **Why is that?**

A   People with type-II diabetes still produce the hormone insulin, but it does not function properly. The problem is tied to being overweight. Generally, someone who is chronically obese has a high carbohydrate intake, and that places a strain on the body's glucose metabolism. At the same time, obesity reduces the body's sensitivity to insulin by causing insulin **receptors** on the surface of the cells to resist insulin. Those cells (primarily muscle and fat cells) then cannot take glucose from the blood, and diabetes results.

In response to the resulting high blood sugar, beta cells in the pancreas struggle to produce more and more insulin. Eventually this overproduction exhausts the beta cells, and insulin secretion becomes inadequate.

Q **Is this what is meant by the term insulin resistance?**
A Doctors often use the term **insulin resistance** to indicate that insulin is present but is not being used efficiently. The reason for insulin resistance is not completely understood, although scientists are striving to learn more about it. Recent research suggests that in some cases it may have to do with the way skeletal muscles store glucose for later use. For us, it's enough to know that insulin resistance plays a role in type-II diabetes.

People with type-II diabetes are often given drugs, called **oral hypoglycaemic agents**, to increase the secretion and effectiveness of insulin. But there's another way to reverse their problems: by cutting back on food intake and losing weight. Apparently, according to various experts, a weight loss of as little as 4.5 to 7 kg (10 to 15 lb) can make a difference in the need for medications to control type-II diabetes.

Q **If I can take drugs for type-II diabetes, then why should I worry about how much sugar I eat?**

A It's true that in type-II diabetes glucose abnormalities may be mild. But that doesn't mean they are any less dangerous. Again, prolonged high blood-sugar levels (hyperglycaemia) – the principal feature of all types of diabetes – damages the body and leads to long-term complications.

Q **Is type-II diabetes easy to spot?**

A Actually, no. This form of diabetes is often hard to detect for several reasons:

- The disease typically exhibits no symptoms for many years, and the onset and progression of symptoms can be slow.
- Typical symptoms are not always present.
- Symptoms are mild and may go unnoticed, which helps explain why there may be millions of people who do not know they have diabetes.

Q **What are the symptoms of type-II diabetes?**

A The symptoms of type-II diabetes are similar to those of type-I, and include the following:

- frequent urination
- increased thirst
- increased hunger
- prolonged and unexplained fatigue
- blurred vision

- numbness or tingling or burning sensations in the legs or feet
- slow-healing wounds or sores
- gynaecological fungal infections in women
- impotence in men.

All too often, however, the symptoms may be very subtle, or they may imitate the symptoms of another disease. And in some cases no symptoms occur at all. It may take years before symptoms manifest themselves.

Q **Then how do people find out that they have type-II?**

A Most people find out they have type-II diabetes when a routine urine test shows sugar, or a blood test reveals high blood-glucose levels. Even a small amount of sugar in the urine is abnormal and should never be ignored. Sometimes the condition is detected when a person visits a doctor to be treated for symptoms of one of the complications of diabetes.

Q **Besides type-I and type-II, what other kinds of diabetes are there?**

A There are several other forms of glucose abnormalities, as doctors often call them. Some of these are not diabetes, but they may signal that diabetes is developing. We will look at four: **increased risk of diabetes**, **impaired glucose tolerance** (IGT), **secondary diabetes** and **gestational diabetes**.

INCREASED RISK OF DIABETES

Q **How is 'increased risk of diabetes' a form of diabetes?**

A Actually, this category is not a form of diabetes, as such. But someone who is classified as being in this group may be at increased risk of developing diabetes one day. Think of this as a warning, urging the person to pay more attention to his or her health.

This type of glucose abnormality includes two categories. The first refers to people with **previous abnormality of glucose tolerance** (formerly called pre-diabetes). People with this have no sign of abnormal glucose metabolism, but they have experienced a period of impaired glucose tolerance or high blood sugar in the past. Women who have had gestational diabetes are also placed in this group.

The second category is called **potential abnormality of glucose**. People who have a close relative with type-I diabetes, or people with islet-cell antibodies, are considered part of this group.

Q **How do doctors treat these people?**

A They don't, because there's really nothing to treat. Doctors should monitor the blood-sugar levels of these people, however, in case something develops down the road.

IMPAIRED GLUCOSE TOLERANCE

Q Impaired glucose tolerance – that's a strange term. What does it mean?

A Glucose tolerance is said to be impaired when blood-sugar levels are higher than normal but not high enough to be diagnosed as diabetes. This impairment is indicated by a fasting-blood-glucose reading between 6.4 and 7.8 mmol/L (115 and 140 mg/dl). Symptoms of diabetes are generally absent.

Q How is this condition related to diabetes?

A Doctors don't consider impaired glucose tolerance a true form of diabetes, but an abnormality in glucose levels – something between normal and 'overt diabetes', as the medical profession terms it. A person who has impaired glucose tolerance may improve, so that blood-sugar levels become normal, or may remain stable, with sugar levels steady in that grey area between normal and high. Perhaps a quarter of people with impaired glucose tolerance go on to develop diabetes.

Q Is impaired glucose tolerance dangerous?

A It doesn't appear that this condition causes severe complications of diabetes, such as kidney failure. But researchers believe that people with impaired glucose tolerance are more likely to have high blood pressure and high **cholesterol** levels – conditions long implicated in coronary heart disease.

SECONDARY DIABETES

Q **What is this?**

A This term is used to describe a host of other conditions that can give rise to diabetes.

Q **Such as?**

A In such cases, the diabetes is secondary to another disease, medication or chemical. Among the causes of secondary diabetes are:

- pancreatic diseases (especially chronic pancreatitis in alcoholics)
- hormonal abnormalities (including those that result from the administration of steroids
- insulin-receptor disorders
- drug- or chemical-induced diabetes
- certain genetic syndromes.

Q **You mean to say that drugs can create a form of diabetes?**

A In some instances, yes, because they increase blood sugar to abnormally high levels.

Q **Which drugs cause this problem, and is the problem permanent or does it go away when the person stops taking the drug?**

A Certain prescription drugs, including glucocorticoids (used as anti-inflammatories), furosemide (a diuretic;

used in blood pressure control), thiazide diuretics (used in blood pressure control), oestrogen-containing products (such as oral contraceptives and hormone-replacement therapy) and beta blockers (used to treat heart disorders) may produce high blood sugar. Any diagnosis of diabetes should take into account the person's history of prescription-drug use.

GESTATIONAL DIABETES

Q Is this a form of diabetes that affects women?

A Yes. Gestational diabetes is any type of diabetes that first appears – or is first recognized – during pregnancy. It develops because of the distinctive hormonal environment and metabolic demands of pregnancy. In 95 per cent of these cases, the diabetes disappears after childbirth.

For some women (about 5 per cent), however, the diabetes remains. And once a woman has had gestational diabetes, she's at risk of developing another form of diabetes (usually type-II) later in life.

Q How many women get gestational diabetes?

A Approximately 3 per cent of pregnant women develop gestational diabetes, but it seems to be more common in women over 25. This age group makes up approximately 50 per cent of all pregnancies but 85 per cent of gestational diabetic pregnancies, according to one medical journal. The risk seems to be similar whether it is a first or subsequent pregnancy.

Q **Is it dangerous?**

A The symptoms of gestational diabetes are generally mild and not life-threatening to the woman. The condition, however, can pose problems for the infant, including hypoglycaemia (low blood sugar) and respiratory-distress syndrome. Women with gestational diabetes are also more susceptible than normal to developing **toxaemia**, a life-threatening condition for both mother and child.

Q **Is gestational diabetes easy to control?**

A Some women find they need to take insulin, but diet and exercise can control gestational diabetes. We talk more about this later in the book.

Q **Again, in general, those symptoms are ...?**

A If you're looking for a rough guideline, here's what the medical literature mentions as important symptoms of untreated or inadequately treated diabetes:

- **Polyuria**: This is the passing of too much urine, or frequent urination.
- Thirst: As you might suspect, polyuria causes dehydration which, in turn, causes thirst.
- Weight loss: The loss of water, as the kidneys strive to eliminate the excess sugar, causes some weight loss. But the main cause of weight loss is the need for the body to use protein and fat to supply the energy that normally would be supplied by properly metabolized glucose. As a result, fat stores and then muscles just waste away.

Tiredness is often present in diabetes, but is not considered a sure symptom since it can be associated with so many other disorders. Other symptoms include unrelenting hunger, itching of the genitals and skin from thrush infections (which thrive on sugar), visual disturbances (such as blurred vision or change of focus), skin disorders (for example, boils) and pain and/or numbness of the extremities.

Q   **Tell me more about the risk of obesity.**

A   As we mentioned earlier, 80 to 85 per cent of people with type-II diabetes are overweight. True, not all overweight people have diabetes, but they could be setting themselves up for this disease 10 or 20 years' hence. As one expert puts it, 'events that occur in middle life (excessive weight gain, for example) can have profound clinical effects 20 years later.'

Q   **What is the definition of 'overweight'?**

A   Definitions vary, but a reasonable one is 'more than 20 per cent over ideal body weight'.

Q   **How about race – is it a risk factor?**

A   The prevalence certainly varies markedly in different countries, but this may have nothing to do with ethnic type. For instance, diabetes is 30 times more common in Scandinavia than it is in Japan. The prevalence also increases steadily as you move from the equator towards the two poles. Countries in order of decreasing risk are: Finland, Sweden, Scotland, Norway, USA,

Denmark, Holland, New Zealand, Canada, England, Poland, France and Japan.

Scientists stress that race alone does not predict diabetes; it must be combined with another factor, such as environmental factors and obesity.

Q **Any other risk factors?**

A Researchers have uncovered a link between poverty and diabetes. Two surveys, conducted by the Gallup Organization in 1989 and in 1990, found a clear relationship between income and diabetes incidence. In the surveys, people with the lowest income had by far the highest incidence of the disease.

Q **What else increases susceptibility to diabetes?**

A A few more factors – some that we've already touched on in this chapter – are:

- being over the age of 40 and having any of the preceding factors
- having impaired glucose tolerance
- having high blood pressure or high cholesterol levels (240 mg/dl or more)
- in women, having a history of gestational diabetes or delivery of babies weighing more than 5 kg (9 lb).

The last of these is a bit misleading; it is not the heavy baby that causes the mother to have diabetes, but the other way round: mothers with diabetes commonly give birth to heavier than normal babies.

Q I see. But, in other words, a person with any one of these risk factors will get diabetes?

A Not necessarily. For the most part, the presence of one risk factor does not predict diabetes, but it does suggest a possibility. The more risk factors you have, the greater your chance of developing diabetes. Apparently, the chances of finding diabetes in someone without a risk factor are low.

Q **How is diabetes diagnosed?**

A At one time, as we suggested, diagnosis consisted of taste-testing the urine. If it was sweet, that was a confirmation of diabetes mellitus. Fortunately, at least for diagnosticians, things are different today. Diabetes is usually confirmed by the typical signs and symptoms, as well as by high glucose levels in the blood and/or urine. In symptomless people, high blood sugar usually is enough for a diagnosis. On the other hand, it is possible for someone to have a little glucose in the urine and not have diabetes, just as it is possible for a person to have mild and moderate elevations in glucose levels but not have diabetes.

When diabetes is suspected, or when a routine blood test reveals high sugar levels – above 11 mmol/L (200 mg/dl), two simple tests are often performed.

Q **Must I go to my doctor for these tests, or can I get a blood-testing kit from the chemist?**

A The diagnosis of diabetes is too important to leave to a self-test kit. This is a job for your doctor. The kits you are thinking of can become very important for you later if, unfortunately, you are found to have diabetes. They are used by people with diabetes to keep track of their day-to-day blood-sugar levels. As a tracking technique, **blood glucose monitoring**, or **BGM** as the medical profession calls it, plays a crucial role in managing diabetes. It gives you the information needed to balance food intake, exercise, and insulin or other medication.

Self-testing is an important aspect of self-care, and we deal with this at some length in Chapter 5. But for now, the major diagnostic tests are performed in a doctor's surgery.

Q OK, then, what are the two simple tests that doctors use, and how do they work?

A The **fasting blood sugar test** is performed after a person hasn't eaten for 8 to 12 hours, usually first thing in the morning. To diagnose diabetes, several of these tests are given on different days. Glucose levels higher than 7.8 mmol/L (140 mg/dl) in two successive tests confirm diabetes.

The **oral glucose-tolerance test** begins with a fasting blood sample taken after a person has eaten an unrestricted high-carbohydrate diet for 3 days. After that sample is taken, the person drinks a glucose solution. Next, blood samples are taken every 30 minutes for two hours, and another sample is taken an hour later. Those blood samples show how the body handles glucose. Normally, blood levels rise after the glucose is drunk and then soon return to normal. In people with diabetes, blood-sugar levels don't fall that quickly. Blood-glucose levels higher than 11 mmol/L (200 mg/dl) 1 to 2 hours after a meal confirm diabetes. If the blood sugar registers over 11 mmol/L (200 mg/dl) after the fasting segment of this test, there's no doubt that the person has diabetes.

Q If doctors can do a blood test at any time to confirm diabetes, isn't there any way to detect it earlier?

A You've put your finger on an important area of diabetes research. Scientists are looking at both diabetes triggers – factors that spark diabetes onset – and diabetes **markers** – genetic signposts, in a manner of speaking. The idea is that, one day, doctors can find those people who will get diabetes and can stop the disease before it starts.

Q What do you mean by a trigger?

A External environmental factors – such as exposure to a virus infection, exposure to certain chemicals or nutritional habits – that trigger an inherited, or genetic, predisposition to diabetes. Scientists think that many different triggers may be responsible for 70 to 95 per cent of type-I cases.

Q Are doctors finding these triggers?

A Yes. One study, reported in 1992, points to cow's milk in infants as an environmental trigger of type-I diabetes. The article notes that 'this study strongly suggests that antibodies to albumin in cow's milk also attack the child's own pancreatic beta cells; thus an immuno-logic reaction to cow's milk may precipitate diabetes in susceptible children.' Based on those findings, the American Academy of Pediatrics recommended that parents *should not* give whole cow's milk to infants under a year of age. In addition, some experts postulate that breastfed infants may be protected against the risk of type-I diabetes later in life.

Q **I've heard a lot lately about genetic research and test-ing. Are there any advances taking place in this area?**

A Doctors and researchers are making headway in identi-fying markers – those genetic indications that a person may develop diabetes.

Q **Such as?**

A One marker appears to be changes in the way the pancreas secretes insulin. Scientists can use special blood tests to identify, with near certainty among first-degree relatives of people with type-I diabetes, those who will develop diabetes. These *assays*, as the tests are called, identify individuals with insulin or islet-cell antibodies.

More research is under way. Other researchers have located two natural tissue **antigens** (substances capable of stimulating the immune system to produce antibod-ies) that serve as markers. These antigens, known as HLA-B8 and HLA-B15, are attacked by the antibodies and white blood cells that make up part of the body's immune system. HLA-B8 and HLA-B15 are more common in peo-ple with type-I diabetes than in people without diabetes.

Q Have there been other advances?

A Researchers have found that a particular pancreatic enzyme stimulates production of antibodies in the blood of many people who eventually develop diabetes. It is not yet clear whether the antibodies play a direct role in destroying insulin-producing cells or whether they are a secondary effect of an autoimmune attack by other cells. In any case, researchers hope that the finding may lead to a simple test to screen for people who are likely to develop the disease, perhaps even years before symptoms appear.

Q What about those of us who already have diabetes?

A Doctors are looking into ways to replace beta cells in the pancreas, primarily through transplantation.

Q Transplantation? You mean surgery that treats diabetes?

A For some people, yes. Today, pancreas transplantation is the only way for people with type-I diabetes to be able to go off insulin. When the pancreas is replaced, the body once again has enough functioning beta cells to produce insulin. The success of pancreas transplants, however, is fairly limited. In 1992, whole pancreas transplants had a 1-year success rate of about 70 per cent and a 5-year success rate of about 50 per cent.

Q Can anyone receive a new pancreas?

A Doctors are currently very selective about pancreatic transplantation. Organ rejection remains the major problem – if the organ you receive does not match your own tissues closely enough, your immune system will attack it. Immunosuppressive drugs help protect the new organ and weaken the rejection response, but they are risky. Because of the risks of the immunosuppressive drugs required for transplantation, many surgeons transplant pancreases only in patients with type-1 diabetes, and only when their kidneys have begun to fail and a kidney transplant is necessary. In that event, of course, immunosuppression is essential, so there is a lot to be said for taking advantage of the opportunity to have a pancreas transplant. The pancreas is transplanted along with a kidney. Anyone interested in pancreatic transplantation should thoroughly discuss the pros and cons with his or her doctor.

Q Will a successful pancreas transplant stop the development of diabetic complications?

A The medical profession is still debating this. Some doctors are enthusiastic. A report from Sweden indicates that kidney disease does not come back in patients who receive both a kidney and pancreas transplant, and German researchers report that the progression of diabetic eye disease is slowed and circulation in the small blood vessels of the legs and feet improves after pancreas transplantation.

Other doctors point out that some complications may already have set in by the time a transplant is indicated, and that the complications will continue despite the new pancreas.

Q This matter of who is eligible for a transplant, and who is likely to do well, is confusing. Where can I go for more information?

A If you're interested in transplantation, we suggest you go to your local library and do some research in the medical journals. Then talk to your doctor.

In addition, the British Diabetes Association (see Sources of Information) can update you on transplantation and where it is being done.

Q What if I'm not eligible for a pancreas transplant or don't want one. Is any other form of surgery available?

A Two other surgical treatments are under investigation:

1 Transplantation of parts of the pancreas – the islets, which contain the beta cells that manufacture insulin. Transplanting the islets can make a person insulin-independent for at least several years. Cell rejection is also still a problem, and so this kind of procedure is still only experimental. Those people who have islet-cell transplants are taking part in the research.

2 A less invasive method of restoring beta cells is also under investigation. Some researchers have been transplanting beta cells, obtained from the pancreas of an adult or a foetus, in people undergoing kidney transplants. Again, cell rejection is a problem with this approach, as is true of any organ replacement.

Q **What about using an artificial pancreas?**

A You may have heard about a device in which beta cells are encapsulated in such a way that the insulin, being small molecules, can get out while the antibodies that would destroy them, being much larger, can't get in. This sounds a wonderful idea, but it is not so easy to achieve success as you might think. As things stand at present, such ideas are experimental and we must wait for progress. At present, most people with diabetes do not expect to have a transplant, and accept that diabetes is something they have to learn to live with.

CHAPTER TWO

INSULIN AND TYPE-1 DIABETES

Q Insulin and type-1 diabetes – do the two always go together?

A Eventually, yes. As we explained in Chapter 1, type-1 diabetes is also known as insulin-dependent diabetes. People with fully-established type-1 diabetes have lost the ability to manufacture the hormone insulin. Thus, they need to receive insulin in the form of injections, to regulate the way their bodies use food for energy.

Some people who are diagnosed as having type-1 diabetes do not immediately require insulin, because their bodies continue to produce small amounts of that hormone. As the disease progresses, however, insulin production stops, and injections are necessary.

Q Can insulin injections cure diabetes?

A Unfortunately, no. Insulin injections merely supply the insulin that the body can't produce. They certainly modify the symptoms of the disease, but they don't treat the cause. In a most basic sense, insulin controls diabetes that cannot be controlled by diet alone. Insulin works *in conjunction* with a disciplined approach to diet – it is not a replacement for proper diet control. If people with diabetes are not careful about the foods they eat and when they eat those foods, they will not be able to control their blood-sugar levels, regardless of insulin intake.

Although this chapter focuses on the role of insulin and how people use it, the fact is that people with type-1 diabetes need both insulin injections and properly regimented diets to stay healthy. Diet is such an important issue for all people with diabetes that we've devoted most of Chapter 5 to the subject.

Q **You've mentioned the words 'discipline' and 'regimented' in conjunction with diet. What do you mean?**

A We mean that most people with diabetes who are insulin dependent lead a fairly structured life. Insulin injections (the most common means of putting insulin into the bloodstream – we discuss others later in this chapter), meals and exercise are carefully scheduled. Even the amount of food and exercise are mapped out in advance. All this structure is necessary to keep blood sugar within a normal range – what the medical profession calls **normoglycaemia** or **euglycaemia**.

You can look at it this way: controlling blood sugar is like walking a narrow path between too much and too little sugar in the blood. Too much (hyperglycaemia) over the years leads to the life-threatening complications touched on in Chapter 1. Blood-sugar levels that are too low (hypoglycaemia) are dangerous because your brain needs an adequate supply of sugar for fuel. Low blood-sugar levels can cause fainting or even death. Eating the right foods, controlling the amount of food you ingest and maintaining the proper amount of insulin in the bloodstream are all essential to keeping well. As we will see, the amount of exercise you take is also an important factor.

Q **Where does insulin come from?**

A There are several kinds or **species** of insulin. **Beef-derived insulin** is obtained from beef pancreases; **pork-derived insulin** comes from pork pancreases. **Human insulin**, a drug chemically identical to the insulin normally produced by the human body, is manufactured in one of two ways: either by using recombinant DNA technology (genetic engineering) or by chemical modification of pork insulin. These two human insulins are known, respectively, as **synthetic** and **semi-synthetic** human insulins.

All insulins come in different forms, each of which acts in a different way.

Q **What are those forms?**

A They are short-acting, intermediate-acting and long-acting. **Short-acting insulins** include acid and neutral soluble preparations. Short-acting insulins are sometimes referred to as fast-acting insulins, as the word *fast* refers to the speed with which the insulin begins to lower blood-sugar levels. Short-acting insulins begin acting in about half an hour and their effect lasts for up to about 8 hours, with a peak effect between 2 and 4 hours after being taken.

Intermediate-acting insulins include biphasic insulins, isophane (**NPH**) insulins and preparations with a predetermined proportion of NPH mixed with soluble, such as 70 per cent NPH to 30 per cent soluble. These begin acting in about an hour and a half and last approximately 12 to 24 hours. **Long-acting insulins** include **PZI** (short for protamine zinc insulin) and insulin zinc suspensions. These begin to take effect in 4 to 6 hours and can last for up to 36 hours.

Q   **So which of these forms are most commonly used by people with type-1 diabetes?**

A   Actually, most people use several forms of insulin. One common approach is to use one form in the morning and another form later in the day. Other people mix insulin forms in the same syringe because they and their doctors have found that mixtures of short-acting with intermediate- or long-acting insulins do a better job of keeping blood-sugar levels normal than does using a single insulin alone. But to answer your question, the most commonly used insulins today are soluble, isophane (NPH), **lente** and **ultralente**.

Because different types of insulin have different pharmacological properties, one form may be preferred over another. Human insulin (Humulin) is recommended for women who are pregnant or considering pregnancy, for people who are allergic to animal-derived insulins, for people who are just beginning insulin

therapy, and for those who must use insulin only inter-
mittently. In fact, most people today are started on
human insulin unless they need PZI, which only comes
in beef-derived form. There is a long-acting Humulin
zinc suspension preparation.

Q **Wait a minute – did I hear you say that a person with
diabetes can be allergic to insulin?**

A Yes. Beef- and pork-derived insulins, the oldest
members of the insulin family, are not identical to
human insulin and can cause allergic reactions around
the spot where the insulin was injected (known as the
injection site).

Q **What kind of allergic reactions do people get?**

A Reactions can range in intensity from a small, red or
itchy area to a widespread skin rash, stomach upset and
even difficulty in breathing. Obviously, this is not something people want to have to put up with. People who
have an allergy to one form of insulin should switch to
another.

Today many animal insulins have been purified,
meaning they are manufactured with fewer impurities,
so allergies are less common. The purest insulins are
the human insulins, made through the high-tech processes mentioned earlier. (Just for the record, today's
animal insulins are 99.99 per cent pure; human insulins
are 99.999 per cent pure!) Since the semi-synthetic
and synthetic human insulins are chemically identical
to the body's own insulin, they do not cause allergic

reactions. More and more people with diabetes are using human insulins.

Q **Are there other differences in insulins?**

A Yes. Insulins vary in three important ways: how quickly the insulin takes effect (doctors use the words **onset** and **absorbency** when talking about this), the intensity of effect or activity it creates (**degree**), and how long the effect lasts (**duration**). For example, human insulins, in general, have a more rapid onset and shorter duration of activity than pork insulins. Beef insulins have the slowest onset and longest duration of activity.

All three of these factors are important, but people with diabetes are often most concerned with onset and absorbency.

Q **Why is that?**

A As we noted, onset and absorbency have to do with when the insulin takes effect. A person with diabetes needs to know when the insulin will start working, because meals are planned around the presence of an appropriate insulin boost. Without that insulin, someone who is insulin-dependent can't absorb and convert sugars into energy.

It's always a challenge to predict accurately how quickly insulin will take effect. A person with diabetes can't be sure insulin will be absorbed at the same rate after each injection. In fact, absorption time differs an average of 25 per cent! Several factors influence how well and how quickly insulin is absorbed.

Q Such as?

A Foremost is the insulin itself. Absorbency differs from manufacturer to manufacturer, even within the same form of insulin. That's why insulin users generally stick to the same brand (manufacturer), the same form (short-, intermediate- or long-acting) and the same species (human, beef, pork) for as long as possible.

    Another important factor – and one that the individual has control over – is the injection site. Insulin is absorbed at different speeds, depending on where it is injected. Injection in the abdomen has the fastest rate of absorption, followed by the arms, thighs and buttocks. Depending upon the person, the lag time for the abdomen might be 30 minutes, while in the thigh it might be 45 minutes. Exercising the arm or leg after injection increases the speed of absorption. In addition, insulin works faster when it is injected in lean areas rather than fat, which is why injection into the buttocks generally offers the slowest absorption rate.

Q Which is better – fast absorption or slow?

A That's entirely up to you and your personal plan. As long as you know the anticipated result, you can calculate when and where to inject your insulin.

Q Sounds a complicated proposition, keeping up with all the factors. Are there any more?

A Yes. Injection techniques, exercise, stress, travelling, hormonal changes (such as menstruation or puberty), and even a person's metabolism affect insulin's onset, degree and duration and, as a result, the blood-sugar levels.

Q **How about the size of the dose – does that matter?**

A Certainly. For a start, dosage varies from person to person. Insulin used to come in concentrations of 40, 100 or 500 units per millilitre (written as U-40, U-100 and U-500). Nowadays, people in Britain nearly all use the U-100 form. This simplifies calculations of dosage and allows standard syringes to be used. The appropriate dose depends on the way an individual's body responds to the planned diet and exercise regimens. Virtually all type-I and many type-II patients need to divide the total daily insulin dosage into 2 or more injections so as to prevent blood-sugar levels from getting too low during the day while maintaining the correct blood-sugar levels through the night.

Q **Now you're going to tell me that, along with everything else a person with diabetes has to contend with, he or she must plan around specific times of the day for the injections. Is that right?**

A Yes. Once again, the best time for an injection depends on blood-sugar levels, food consumption, exercise and the forms of insulin used.

Generally, doctors recommend an interval of 30 minutes between injection of short-acting insulin and a meal. They discourage people from eating within a few minutes after (or before) injecting short-acting insulin, because that substantially reduces the insulin's ability to prevent a rapid rise in blood sugar and, thus, increases the risk of low blood sugar (hypoglycaemia) a few hours later. The person and his or her GP can set up guidelines for the suggested interval between insulin injection and mealtime based on factors such as blood-sugar levels, site of injection and anticipated activity during the interval.

Q **I'm worried. This is a lot of information to have to juggle at one time. Is there anything that can help to make this juggling act easier?**

A Yes. Your doctor should set up a daily treatment plan, which spells out elements such as dosage, insulin concentration, type of syringe and timing of injections.

He or she should also prepare an **algorithm** for a patient with diabetes – a simple 'if this, then do that ... if not this, then do that' type of mathematical chart which can serve as a guide for determining how many units of insulin to take and when to take them, depending upon blood-sugar level. There's one hitch to using an algorithm, however.

Q **And what's that?**

A The person must regularly test his or her blood-glucose levels.

Q **What kind of test?**

A This regular testing is called self-monitoring of blood glucose, or BGM. We mentioned it briefly in Chapter 1, and we discuss it in depth in Chapter 5. Quite simply, it's a way of monitoring blood-sugar fluctuations throughout the day, so that the person with diabetes can do a better job of reaching target blood-sugar levels.

Q How would I do self-monitoring?

A You use a blood-glucose meter (available on prescription from your doctor) to measure the blood-sugar level in a drop of your blood. The test takes 45 seconds to 2 minutes to give results. With the blood-glucose measurement literally in hand, you then look at your algorithm for guidance on how many units of insulin to inject.

The algorithm is a handy tool. If you don't have one, ask your doctor to create one. Because each algorithm varies from person to person, you can't follow anyone else's. An algorithm also needs constant reassessment and occasional updating, since diabetes is a disease that doesn't stay still. From time to time, you and your doctor may find that a change in species or brand of insulin may be necessary to keep pace with the current status of your disease, or perhaps with new and more valuable formulations of insulin.

Q What about that insulin? Are there certain things that I should be looking for when getting my insulin from the chemist?

A The most important step is to double-check the bottles to be sure you are getting the correct type, strength and brand. This is particularly important if you purchase pre-mixed insulins, because they can be prepared in all sorts of combinations.

Pharmacists must not change your insulin preparations in any way without your doctor's approval – or without informing you – but mix-ups can happen. When you go for your insulin, take along an empty bottle. Or keep a copy of a label to help you verify that you have the right stuff.

Finally, check the expiry date before you leave the shop. Will you be able to use all the insulin before it expires? If not, ask for another bottle with a later shelf date.

Q How often must I use insulin?

A The answer depends upon what blood-sugar levels you and your doctor are trying to maintain. Basically, there are two types of diabetes therapy. The first is known as the **standard** or **conventional therapy**. It's been used for decades.

The second, newer therapy is called **tight control** or **intensive therapy**. As the names imply, this therapy strives for tighter control of blood-sugar levels, and generally that means striving for less fluctuation in sugar levels.

Q Which therapy is better?

A We wish there was a definite answer, but you've put your finger on one of the most hotly debated aspects of diabetes care today. Doctors hold a confusing range of positions for and against tight control. We'll see why in a moment. The matter is one of great importance on which decisions must not be made lightly. The arguments on both sides are cogent.

To settle at least part of the debate, a group of doctors and scientists are conducting a large research trial to investigate the merits of tight control. Known as the Diabetes Control and Complications Trial, this project gives a definition of tight control, which we use in this book. Basically, they define a tight-control regimen as one in which people with diabetes strive to maintain near-normal blood-sugar levels by either going on an **insulin pump** (we'll talk about this shortly) or by taking 4 to 6 insulin injections daily and performing at least 4 self-administered tests of blood-glucose levels per day.

Q **How different is that regimen from standard treatment?**

A Standard diabetes treatment generally entails 2 insulin injections a day. The **mixed-split regimen** (mixtures of intermediate-acting and short-acting insulin given before breakfast and dinner) is the most commonly used conventional scheme. Along with this comes self-monitoring of blood glucose once or twice a day.

The advantage of standard treatment is that it's a fairly easy routine to follow. The drawback is that it's fairly inflexible. Once you take your morning insulin, for instance, you can't change the time of your meals or their size — at least not without throwing blood-sugar levels out of the desired range. It's difficult to make spur-of-the-moment changes and still keep blood sugar under control.

Q **So is that why an intensive therapy of tight control was developed – to remedy some of the drawbacks of standard treatment?**

A Generally speaking, yes. One of the goals of tight control is to make the diabetes treatment programme more responsive to a person's lifestyle, rather than changing a lifestyle to fit the treatment programme. With the technique of tight control, a person with diabetes takes more frequent, smaller injections of insulin each day. As a result, he or she has a great deal more flexibility in the timing of meals and exercise. Many doctors believe that when patients have more flexibility, they are more likely to follow a treatment approach.

A second goal of the intensive, tight-control therapy is to achieve better control over blood-sugar levels, so as to maintain more stable sugar levels and reduce the incidence of complications. This will work if you are willing to invest a lot of time and energy in a demanding routine of frequent injections and blood tests day after day after day. Many people feel physically better with a tight-control regimen, and they like the sense of empowerment they gain from being able to keep their blood sugar within a narrow range. For them, the feeling and sense of power are worth the extra effort. Most of all, there is the awareness that they are getting somewhere near the kind of blood sugar fluctuations experienced by a person who does not have diabetes. And people who do not have diabetes do not develop diabetic complications.

Q But you said that tight control is controversial. Why is that if the regimen helps people feel better and the results are so good?

A For one thing, many people with diabetes don't want to devote that much effort to managing their disease. They are used to the standard regimen of 2 injections a day, and they don't want to spend more time testing their blood-sugar levels and injecting insulin more frequently.

But the big concern and the source of much of the controversy with tight control is that blood-sugar levels can get too low, leading to hypoglycaemia. Also known as an **insulin reaction** or a low blood-glucose attack, hypoglycaemia is caused by too much insulin in the bloodstream. As we mentioned in Chapter 1, early symptoms of hypoglycaemia include trembling, hunger, weakness and irritability. If blood glucose drops too low, a person may pass out, go into a coma and could even die.

Q What factors can cause low blood sugar?

A Several things can provoke hypoglycaemia:

- delaying or skipping a meal
- not eating enough carbohydrates in a meal
- sudden increase in amount of exercise
- taking too much insulin.

We talk more about hypoglycaemia and how to treat it in Chapter 4. But for now, it's enough to say that it's a situation people need to avoid.

Q   **Are you saying that people on tight control are more likely to get hypoglycaemia?**

A   Yes. That is what the experts are saying. As early as 1990, the Diabetes Control and Complications Trial reported that people following an intensive therapy of tight control were three times more likely to experience severe hypoglycaemia – in other words, reactions so intense that they required the assistance of another person to recover.

Q   **If this can happen, then why do doctors support tight control?**

A   Many doctors, including some diabetes specialists, stand squarely behind tight control, in spite of the likelihood of hypoglycaemia. Proponents argue that patients on tight control can achieve admirably low and stable blood-sugar levels. They also point out that the research has not demonstrated that frequent bouts of hypoglycaemia pose long-term hazards. And they see tight control as the preferable approach until science comes up with a better treatment for diabetes.

Q   **So what's the argument against tight control?**

A   Opponents of tight control claim that it is potentially dangerous with no proven benefit, that it is far too labour-intensive for both patient and doctor, that it is expensive to implement. These views were expressed by one of the principal investigators in the Diabetes Control and Complications Trial. This expert has advised that doctors should be cautious about using intensive therapies until the results of the trial are fully known. His greatest concern was that doctors who are not experienced in managing intensive therapy may encounter an even greater risk-to-benefit ratio than that documented by the trial so far.

For those reasons, many doctors are taking a wait-and-see approach. If some of their patients request intensive therapy, they may cautiously tighten control. But for the time being they continue to advocate average control until more data are released. One thing is certain: *Never* attempt to switch to tight control on your own initiative. Do it only with the full knowledge, approval and co-operation of your doctor.

Q **Let's say I start a tight-control regimen, with frequent doses of insulin. Do I have to worry about drug interactions?**

A As a well-informed person, you should discuss potential drug interactions any time you take more than one medication, be it a prescription drug or an over-the-counter preparation. Even aspirin, cold remedies, antacids, laxatives and smoking deterrents (such as nicotine patches or chewing gum) may affect the way insulin works, so that your dose of insulin may have to be adjusted. When in doubt about interactions, ask. When not in doubt, ask yourself why not!

Q **What if I'm ill? Do I stop taking insulin?**

A The answer is a most emphatic *no*. But illness can change the effect of insulin. Most of the time you'll need to take more insulin; in some cases you may be able to reduce your insulin dose. It's essential that you call your doctor for instructions on adjusting your treatment. Blood sugar can skyrocket during an illness, especially if you have a cold, flu, infection or injury.

Q **Some people have told me to keep my insulin in the fridge; other people tell me not to. What's best?**

A Most practitioners recommend that you keep your insulin bottle at room temperature, because cold insulin can be painful when injected and may not be absorbed as well. Insulin remains stable – in other words, usable and effective – up to 3 months without refrigeration.

A few practitioners, however, recommend that you refrigerate the bottle you're currently using. Their advice is based on evidence that unrefrigerated insulin sometimes loses potency after the bottle has been in use for more than 30 days. The loss in potency is slight, which is why most doctors don't believe that refrigeration is necessary.

All the experts do agree on two things: people with diabetes should have on hand a spare bottle of each type of insulin used, and that vials of insulin *not in use* should be refrigerated. But don't freeze them, and be sure to keep them away from heat and direct sunlight.

Q **How can I tell if insulin has lost its potency?**

A There are a few obvious indicators:

- The expiry date has passed. If so, open a new bottle.

- The bottle has been open and unrefrigerated for more than 3 months. If you store insulin at room temperature, write the date on the bottle when you open it.
- The insulin looks different. Inspect insulin before you use it. Has it changed in colour or clarity? In general, short-acting insulin is clear and other insulins are uniformly cloudy. Is there sediment at the bottom of the bottle? Have small lumps or clumps formed? A yes answer to any one question signals a loss in potency.

Q **OK, I've checked my insulin and it looks fine. How do I load the syringe?**

A Talk to your GP about the fine points of technique; injection methods are best demonstrated face-to-face. In addition, re-read the instruction sheet that you should have received when you purchased your insulin and syringes.

But to answer your question, we'll review a few basics: clean your hands and the injection site before each injection. Wipe the top of the insulin vial with 70 per cent isopropyl alcohol. For all insulin preparations except short-acting, the vial should be gently rolled in the palms of the hands (not shaken) to re-suspend the insulin. Don't shake it – that might cause loss of potency. After the insulin is drawn into the syringe, check the insulin for air bubbles. Give the top of the upright syringe one or two quick flicks with your forefinger to encourage air bubbles to escape.

Bubbles decrease the size of the dose.

Ask for help if you're not feeling confident about using a syringe, because improper cleansing or injection technique may lead to an infection.

Q   **Can I re-use syringes?**

A   If you have glass syringes, you must sterilize them first before re-using them. If you're asking about re-using disposable syringes – well, that's another issue debated in the medical world. Disposable syringes and needles are made for one use. Manufacturers won't guarantee the sterility of re-used syringes. But since the cost of disposable syringes and needles really adds up over the course of a year, many people prefer to re-use a syringe until its needle becomes dull.

Q   **Is that a safe thing to do?**

A   Some authorities do not recommend re-using syringes and needles. Others acknowledge that syringe re-use appears both safe and practical for many people with diabetes. The reason, they say, is that most insulin preparations contain additives that inhibit the growth of bacteria commonly found on the skin.

Q   **If I'm supposed to wipe the top of the insulin vial with 70 per cent isopropyl alcohol, should I also clean the needle with alcohol?**

A   Some doctors recommend that you wipe the needle with alcohol after each use. Others argue that using alcohol to cleanse the needle offers no clear benefit, adding that alcohol may remove the needle's silicon coating and, thus, make injection more painful.

Q **Personally, I hate needles. Are there alternatives to syringes?**

A Many people with diabetes accept syringes as part of their self-care, while others have difficulty overcoming their distaste of needles. The good news is that a host of alternative devices for delivering insulin are available or in development. Let's look at some of them.

INSULIN PUMPS

Q **What is an insulin pump?**

A Insulin infusion pumps, as they are more precisely called, are small, battery-operated devices that pump insulin into the body at specified intervals. They include a small mechanical motor; a display window for reading measurements; a battery; a small supply of insulin (enough for several days); and a small tube, or **catheter**, connected to a needle through which the insulin flows under the skin. Insulin pumps often have a little numerical keyboard for controlling the amount of insulin that gets dispensed.

Worn on a belt or strapped to the body, pumps release insulin at frequent, pre-scheduled times. Today's pumps are programmable, meaning that the pump-wearer can programme the pump to deliver less insulin during the period when blood sugar is likely to be down (usually the middle of the night) and more insulin for those times when blood sugar tends to rise (usually early in the morning – what is called the **dawn phenomenon**).

In medical language, therapy with an infusion pump is called **continuous subcutaneous insulin infusion** (CSII). Insulin pump management is still too new for general use but is being used by patients under the care of diabetes specialists or diabetes clinics. It really requires the guidance of a skilled professional team, including a doctor experienced in CSII therapy, capable of providing continuous care in case problems should develop.

Q **Aside from avoiding syringes, what are the advantages of using an infusion pump?**

A In some patients, pumps and CSII provide the same kind of improvement in blood-sugar control as multiple insulin injections (the 'tight control' we spoke about earlier). And insulin pumps, like frequent injections, provide more flexibility about mealtimes. The user can also programme in an extra burst of insulin if needed.

Q **Can anyone use an infusion pump?**

A Some doctors recommend CSII only when 3 or 4 daily injections fail to control blood sugar. But other doctors see it as a matter of personal choice. The best candidates are people who are strongly motivated to improve their sugar levels, and who have the discipline to monitor their blood-sugar levels regularly through self-testing.

Q **There must be some disadvantages in pump therapy. What's the bad news?**

A Like any therapy based on a mechanical device, pump therapy can pose a few potential complications, and anyone who uses an infusion pump needs to be aware of them. For instance, undetected interruptions in insulin delivery may result in episodes of extremely high blood sugar, which is why frequent blood-sugar tests are essential. Infections or inflammation at the needle site are other potential complications; they can be minimized by careful hygiene and by changing the needle site frequently.

Then there's the issue of appearance, which is more important to some people than others. Although infusion pumps come in various sizes, most of them are about the size of a mobile phone and weigh about 180g (6 oz). They are worn in a pouch on a waist or shoulder belt and are battery-operated. The best models incorporate an alarm that sounds on malfunction.

Q **Will pumps be getting smaller and less conspicuous?**

A Manufacturers are making them smaller every year. But for the most inconspicuous pump of all, the award goes to the newest development in pump therapy: the **implantable pump**, also known as the **closed-loop pump**. This small device, which is inserted under the skin, is still in clinical trial and is not yet available to the average patient.

Q **How is an implantable pump supposed to work?**

A The implanted pump is a complete unit inserted within the body, often around the abdomen. There are no long tubes or view windows, because these little computerized pumps decide how much insulin is needed and then automatically release it. In theory, they closely imitate the insulin actions of the pancreas.

Q **I recall hearing about problems with implants. Have they been resolved?**

A According to an article in the *New England Journal of Medicine*, implanted pumps had plenty of problems in clinical trials during the early 1980s. Insulin tended to collect within the pump or catheter, batteries had a short life, and mechanical failures were frequent. Most of these problems seem to have disappeared in the implanted pumps of the 1990s. Catheter blockages are still the most common complication, but they can be overcome by changing the catheter under local anaesthetic.

Q **These sound very promising. Are there any other drawbacks?**

A Unfortunately, implanted pumps have a rather short lifespan – 15 to 30 months, according to several pilot studies. For the time being, at least, they are not a means of lifelong insulin delivery.

JET INJECTORS

Q How do these devices work?

A   As the name implies, jet injectors use pressure to shoot insulin into the skin with jetlike speed. A little larger than a syringe, jet injectors have no needles. Thus, they are particularly useful devices for adults who are so frightened by needles that they don't take insulin as often as directed.

Jet injection is not exactly new: it was first proposed for use with insulin in the 1950s. Today's injectors appear to be mechanically reliable and accurate. Compared with syringe injection, insulin absorption and distribution differ when administered by jet injection. In general, jet-injected insulin causes a larger drop in blood sugar than an equal amount of insulin administered by syringe – meaning that less insulin is needed to do the job.

Q Do they have any drawbacks?

A   Some people complain that jet injectors are cumbersome to sterilize, while others point out that jet injection is not necessarily less painful than a needle. A few doctors are still worried about the consistency of the delivered insulin dose, but on the whole jet injectors have an established place among the ranks of insulin-delivery devices.

INSULIN PENS

Q **How do insulin pens work?**

A Like syringes, insulin pens use needles to inject insulin. But instead of having to handle vials of insulin, the user simply pops in a cartridge of insulin, indicates the appropriate number of units of insulin, and shoots the insulin in.

As the name suggests, these devices are shaped like pens. Disposable needles attach at one end. Insulin pens are popular with people who take multiple daily injections of insulin, as in the intensive, or tight-control, regimen.

Q **What of the future?**

A Researchers are talking about developing an insulin pill, and some predict that the day is coming when people may take insulin through an eyedropper. But both these concepts are still under study, and results won't be seen for many years. There is also the possibility, already mentioned, of maintaining donor islet cells in antibody-protected capsules so that they can monitor blood-sugar levels and secrete insulin. Diabetes is an area in which intensive research and new ideas abound. There is so much to be gained, both for patients and for those commercially involved, that you can be sure that if major advances are possible, they will happen.

CHAPTER THREE

TYPE-II DIABETES

Although this chapter is concerned primarily with type-II diabetes, a good deal of what is in it applies equally to long-term type-I diabetes. You should bear this in mind while reading it.

Q **Which is the more serious condition, type-I diabetes or type-II diabetes?**

A The one thing both forms of diabetes have in common is high blood sugar, and that's serious regardless of how it comes about.

However, type-I diabetes is considered to be more severe, primarily because it arises swiftly and can be life-threatening. As you may recall from Chapter 1, type-I diabetes is caused when the pancreas does not produce insulin. Since the body needs insulin to turn food into energy, people with type-I diabetes absolutely must take insulin in order to live. That's why they are called insulin-dependent. Without insulin, these people will develop ketoacidosis, a deadly build-up of poisons in the blood-stream that can occur in a matter of days.

Q **So do those of us with type-II diabetes have to worry?**

A Yes. Type-II diabetes is also hazardous. It just poses a different sort of danger, to long-term health.

By now, you know that people with type-II diabetes still have the ability to produce some insulin, but usually not enough. In addition, the insulin they do produce no longer functions properly. People with type-II diabetes are called non-insulin-dependent, even though many of them eventually rely on insulin, at least for a time, to manage their disease.

Q **So how is this dangerous?**

A Type-II diabetes accounts for 85 to 90 per cent of all cases of diabetes. Working with all these people has given the medical profession plenty of time to find out about the long-term characteristics of this disease. And they have found that type-II is more insidious — meaning that it can proceed undetected for many years. Scientists estimate that the period from the onset of type-II diabetes to its diagnosis can vary from 4 to 12 years. Because the symptoms are not dramatic, no one notices its presence. Unfortunately, in that time the high sugar levels associated with the diabetes may have set the stage for some serious problems, particularly heart disease and circulatory problems. Someone with diabetes, for example, is twice as likely to have a history of heart attack or stroke than his or her peers who do not have diabetes. In fact, the longer someone has the disease, the greater the risk of experiencing a related illness.

Q **Do many people with type-II diabetes get a related illness?**

A Unfortunately, yes. Long-term diabetes, whether type-I or type-II, is often very bad news. Approximately one person in 250 becomes seriously disabled from the disease each year, mainly from heart attacks, strokes, bleeding inside the eyes, kidney disorders and loss of the blood supply to the limbs. These complications occur because diabetes damages the arteries, causing hardening, narrowing and partial obstruction. So any of the organs or parts supplied by these arteries can be damaged. So far as the extremities are concerned, diabetic arterial disease can lead to gangrene and the need for amputation.

Q **Strokes, heart attacks, hardening of the arteries, amputations – these sound like problems of the elderly, no?**

A Yes, many of the complications of diabetes are the same as those associated with advanced age, because many of these misfortunes are the result of artery disease. People with long-term diabetes of whichever type are just that much more likely to develop arterial disease. All this is evidence of what we've noted before – that diabetes hastens the wear and tear on many crucial bodily functions and that good control of blood-sugar levels is vital.

Q Do all people with long-term diabetes experience this wear and tear?

A To greatly varying degrees, yes. But by scrupulous attention to a healthy lifestyle and a strong commitment to maintaining target blood-sugar levels, people with diabetes can usually significantly slow down the degenerative process. There are a lucky few who have their blood sugar in such control that it's almost as though they no longer have the disease.

Sad to say, however, there are no complete guarantees. Someone may be a model of self-care and discipline yet still experience a major complication; another person who has always had wildly swinging sugar levels may live to a ripe old age. These, however, are the exceptions. Much research has shown that good control does work. All the experts are adamant: the time a person with diabetes spends on self-care does indeed help to minimize complications.

Q So what can you tell me about the mechanics of type-II diabetes?

A The more the medical world studies type-II diabetes, the more scientists learn that it works in various ways. Scientists now think type-II diabetes has several components:

- an inability of the pancreas to produce insulin
- an abnormal production of glucose by the liver
- insulin resistance, or a problem with the way insulin functions in the body.

Q Do all people with type-II diabetes have all these components?

A Not necessarily. An individual may have one, two or three, but the most common component by far is insulin resistance. Virtually all people with type-II have this form of metabolic malfunction.

INSULIN RESISTANCE

Q What, again, is insulin resistance exactly?

A Insulin resistance is a term used to describe the situation when the pancreas makes insulin, but for some reason the insulin is not very effective at transferring glucose from the blood into the cells of the body. Imagine your cells as little orbs powered by that form of sugar known as glucose. On the surface of these orbs are tiny structures, called receptors, that serve as gateways into the cell. In order for a cell to absorb glucose, its gateways must be open. Insulin is the hormone that opens these gates by latching onto the cell at its **receptor sites**.

Several problems can develop in people with type-II diabetes. First, the number of receptors on each cell is lower than normal. Second, some of the insulin is not able to latch on to the receptor sites – in effect, these people's cells are resistant to their body's insulin. Third, the pancreas' insulin-producing capacity declines.

Q   So if I understand you correctly, you're saying that people with type-II diabetes have plenty of insulin in their bodies?

A   Not necessarily, but very often. People with type-II diabetes may have normal or even above-normal levels of insulin.

Q   **Above normal? How does that happen?**

A   Think of those beta cells in the pancreas, trained to respond whenever blood sugar goes above a certain level. When blood-sugar levels build up because insulin isn't doing its job well, the beta cells cheerfully pump out more insulin. But still that insulin doesn't get used efficiently.

In some people, a high level of insulin eventually builds up in the blood – a situation doctors call **hyperinsulinaemia**.

Q   **Is it a problem?**

A   This is something doctors wonder about. It has been suggested that insulin itself may contribute over the long term to disease of the arteries – in other words, the condition known as **atherosclerosis**. But many doctors point out that this concern is purely speculative, with little supporting evidence.

Q   **Why do people develop these insulin problems in the first place?**

A   Scientists have linked type-II diabetes to two predisposing factors. The first is heredity.

HEREDITY

Q   **Are you saying that type-II diabetes is hereditary?**

A   Yes. Type-II diabetes often runs in families, suggesting that some genetic trait puts people at greater risk of developing type-II diabetes.

Q   **Do doctors have any idea of what that genetic trait may be?**

A   Well, yes. A recent article in the *New England Journal of Medicine* hypothesized that a defect in the way in which skeletal muscles convert glucose into **glycogen** (the form in which glucose is stored for later use) may underlie the development of type-II diabetes.

We need to focus on one key point: you are not born with insulin resistance or type-II diabetes – but you may be born with the ability to develop type-II diabetes. And this leads us straight to the next influencing factor – obesity.

OBESITY

Q   **What is obesity?**

A   Being overweight. Intimately related to this is overeating, which in and of itself can exacerbate type-II diabetes. In fact, obesity is considered to be the primary trigger for insulin resistance and type-II diabetes. Approximately 85 per cent of people with type-II diabetes are obese

(20 per cent or more over their ideal body weight) and, in almost all cases, the obesity preceded the development of overt diabetes.

Q   **Do all overweight people eventually develop diabetes?**
A   No, although many of them become insulin-resistant, even though they don't develop the skyrocketing sugar levels seen with diabetes. Being overweight places heavy demands on the body for more insulin and contributes to insulin resistance. A person who might need about 50 units of insulin a day at a normal weight might require as much as 120 units daily to maintain normal blood sugar when overweight.

Again, some researchers argue that insulin resistance is an acquired condition, not one that people are born with. Some go so far as to argue that obesity is the disease and diabetes the complication. Whether or not you agree with this view, researchers have found that both insulin resistance and type-II diabetes can be reversed to a great extent by successful weight loss.

Q   **Do you mean that diabetes can be treated through diet?**
A   Yes. Diet has been called the cornerstone of treatment for type-II diabetes. It's generally the first treatment a person with diabetes tries.

DIET

Q   **What kind of diet?**

A   *Diet* is a tricky word. On the one hand, it means careful attention to the foods you eat. On the other hand, the word conjures up images of short-term, intensive periods of calorie deprivation which may or may not be nutritionally sound. What most diabetes experts mean by diet is a carefully composed eating plan – a plan that someone with diabetes can comfortably continue for life. This eating plan might be developed with the assistance of a dietitian. It will address not only how much food can be eaten but also the types of food to eat. Following an eating plan to improve blood sugar is known as **diet therapy**.

Q   **What does it entail?**

A   Diet therapy includes two strategies: calorie control and weight loss. For most people with diabetes, accomplishing both requires a complete change in eating habits – a new way of thinking about food, in effect. We discuss the particulars of nutrition for people with diabetes in Chapter 5.

Q   **What can a new eating plan achieve?**

A   For someone with type-II diabetes who is not overweight, simply controlling calories may be all that is needed to improve blood-sugar levels markedly. In someone who is overweight, the weight loss achieved with a low-calorie diet can produce a major improvement in blood-sugar levels.

The moment someone stops overeating, the need for insulin decreases and insulin production slows. Remember that insulin production is stimulated each time food is eaten.

Cutting back on food intake can immediately reduce blood-glucose levels. At the same time, the symptoms of diabetes – hunger and thirst, fatigue, frequent urination – begin to lessen within a few days, and even before the person has lost an ounce of weight!

Q   **Why does this happen so quickly?**

A   It's theorized that proper diet helps insulin receptors work more effectively. In a sense, they're not constantly being overwhelmed by calories.

Q   **You've been talking about using diet to lower blood-glucose levels. Just what kind of blood-glucose figures should people with diabetes aim for?**

A   Targets vary from person to person. Some doctors set a narrower or slightly different range from what we're showing here, according to their own standards of practice. But as a rule of thumb, targets include blood glucose in the range of 3.8 to 6.6 mmol/L (70 to 120 mg/dl) in the morning before eating; 10 to 11 mmol/L (180 to 200 mg/dl) 1 hour after a meal; and 3.8 to 7.2 mmol/L (70 to 130 mg/dl) 3 hours after a meal. These are much lower blood-glucose levels than were aimed at years ago.

Again, targets snould vary. Each person with diabetes and his or her doctor must work together towards setting realistic goals.

Q How much weight does someone need to lose to see blood-sugar improvements?

A Not as much as you might think. A 10 per cent weight loss is the figure we've most often come across. Depending upon the individual's weight, that may mean as little as 10 pounds. As one doctor puts it, the goal of weight loss is to decrease insulin resistance, and a person with diabetes doesn't always have to reach his or her ideal weight to improve blood-sugar levels. The point is, any amount of weight loss is good, because it immediately decreases the amount of insulin you need.

Q Besides consuming fewer calories, are there other things a person with type-II diabetes has to do related to diet?

A Actually, yes. Many people with type-II diabetes also have **hypertension** (high blood pressure) and **hyperlipidaemia** (a high level of fat in the blood). Both hypertension and hyperlipidaemia are associated with an increased risk of heart disease – just what you don't need. In addition, high blood pressure strains the heart, damages the arteries and increases the risk of stroke, heart attack and kidney problems.

Hypertension and hyperlipidaemia are both affected by the type of foods people eat. In Chapter 5, we discuss the foods that should be avoided to keep blood pressure and blood fats down.

Q How many people control diabetes solely by diet?

A Not enough, unfortunately. Statistics paint a rather sobering picture: at the end of 1 year, only 10 to 20 per cent of people with type-II diabetes are able to bring their blood-glucose levels down to normal through diet. Within 5 years of diagnosis of their disease, around 90 per cent with type-II diabetes need another treatment method.

Q Why is the success rate so low?

A It could be that the success rate would be much higher if more people with diabetes combined a change in eating habits with an earnest commitment to exercise. The medical books often list exercise as being the second step in the treatment of type-II diabetes, but ideally it should be part and parcel of diet therapy.

Q Why is exercise important?

A Exercise itself helps reduce blood-glucose levels and makes insulin more effective. Exercise also helps people lose weight faster. And it helps them maintain their lower weight.

There are other suspected benefits. Exercise seems to improve insulin's sensitivity (its ability to work), reduces the dosage required or the need for blood-glucose-reducing medications, and reduces the risk of cardiovascular disease. Exercise is recommended for everyone – with or without diabetes. We discuss it at greater length in Chapter 5.

Q   **Can people control their diabetes simply by getting lots of exercise? Wouldn't that make all the concern about diet unnecessary?**

A   No. Exercise alone can't control blood-sugar levels, except in rare cases. Some people think that as long as they are exercising vigorously and regularly, they can eat as much of anything they want. Wrong! Exercise won't control blood glucose, although it does influence it. As we said before, a sound meal plan forms the cornerstone of all treatment for type-II diabetes. Everything else must build on that sound base.

ORAL THERAPY

Q   **What if exercise and diet don't reduce my blood sugar? What's next?**

A   If meal planning, better eating habits, weight loss and regular exercise do not keep your blood sugar within your target range, then most GPs recommend using drugs to lower blood glucose. Referred to as oral hypoglycaemic agents, oral hypoglycaemics or oral agents, these pills are also prescribed for those people who (for whatever reason) are unable or unwilling to control their weight and food intake. The use of these pills is called **oral therapy**.

Q **What do these drugs do?**

A Oral hypoglycaemics lower blood-sugar levels. They seem to do it by increasing the amount of insulin the pancreas secretes and by helping the body use that insulin more effectively.

Q **What kind of oral hypoglycaemic agents are available?**

A Oral agents come from two chemical families, the **sulphonylureas** and the **biguanides**.

Q **Tell me about them.**

A The sulphonylureas were developed after it was noted in the 1940s that the then-widely used sulpha drugs caused a drop in blood sugar. Derivatives of the sulphonamides, tolbutamide and chlorpropamide, were introduced in 1956 and 1957 respectively. These drugs work mainly by forcing the islet cells of the pancreas to produce more insulin. They are, of course, useless in people with type-I diabetes, whose islet cells have been destroyed. They also help by increasing the number of insulin receptors on cells.

The second class, the biguanides, were discovered in 1967. They work by reducing absorption of carbohydrates from the intestine, reducing the rate at which the liver synthesizes glucose and increasing the ability of muscle cells to take up glucose.

Q **What are their names?**

A There are quite a number of them. The sulphonylureas include:

- **tolbutamide** (Rastinon)
- **tolazamide** (Tolanase)
- **glibenclamide** (Daonil, Euglucon)
- **chlorpropamide** (Diabinase)
- **gliclazide** (Diamicron)
- **glipizide** (Glibenese, Minodiab)
- **gliquidone** (Glurenorm).

The only biguanide commonly prescribed in Britain is **metformin** (Glucophage).

Q   **If I decide to use an oral hypoglycaemic, how frequently would I take it?**

A   This is not a decision you should take for yourself. These drugs are potentially dangerous and can cause hypoglycaemia. You must discuss this with your doctor. When you do, you will learn that some oral agents must be taken more than once a day; others can be taken only once daily. Your doctor will set up a schedule for you.

Q   **Can people with type-I diabetes use oral hypoglycaemics?**

A   No. Oral hypoglycaemics work only if the body's beta cells are already producing some insulin. Because the beta cells in people with type-I diabetes have been irrevocably destroyed, these drugs can do nothing for them.

Q Can these drugs be used for all people with type-II diabetes?

A You bring up an important point – oral hypoglycaemics work better on some people than others. They work best on people who develop diabetes after the age of 40, whose disease is newly discovered and who take less than 40 units of insulin a day. In prescribing oral hypoglycaemics, doctors take into account the person's age, weight and overall health. Oral agents aren't recommended for pregnant women, because the effect on the foetus is not known.

Q When someone takes oral hypoglycaemics, does he or she still have to be careful about what she eats?

A If you mean, 'Does he or she have to control calorie intake and eat the right foods?' the answer is 'Absolutely yes.' Diet can make or break the success of oral therapy. These drugs won't work if the eating plan is neglected. It's not just a matter of increasing the dosage to make up for eating too much: Beyond the recommended maximum dosage, oral hypoglycaemics are not any more potent or effective.

Someone with diabetes needs to be careful not to get lulled into a false sense of security just because the blood sugar has suddenly improved thanks to the pills. No one with diabetes can safely neglect the eating plan and exercise programme or skip blood-sugar monitoring. Oral hypoglycaemics do not replace a healthy lifestyle.

Q   **Presumably these drugs do have their disadvantages. What are they?**

A   A very important one, for a start, we have already hinted at: anyone who uses oral hypoglycaemic agents is at risk of developing very low blood-glucose levels, a situation known as hypoglycaemia. Symptoms of hypoglycaemia include hunger, sweating, shaking, dizziness, confusion, irritability, even nausea.

Anyone who begins oral therapy must monitor blood-sugar levels several times a day initially. Once the person has got accustomed to these drugs and has brought blood glucose into the target range, he or she may be able to schedule blood-glucose measurements once a day or once every other day. The thing to watch for is a blood-glucose level of 3.4 mmol/L (60 mg/dl) or below. At that point, the patient needs to take steps *immediately* to get blood-sugar levels higher. Eating certain foods or injecting glucose are two ways to do this; see Chapter 4 for complete details.

Q   **Besides the possibility of low blood sugar, are there other problems with oral hypoglycaemic agents?**

A   Yes. Another common occurrence is allergic reaction. A rash, hives, nausea, vomiting or cramping may be a sign of an allergy. If so, the doctor may prescribe a different oral hypoglycaemic. These drugs also tend to react in a strange way with alcohol. The combination of the two may create a reaction that includes an excruciating headache, a flushed face and nausea. Although usually harmless, this reaction can be quite startling and is occasionally dangerous. Again, a different oral agent may not cause this reaction.

Q **Speaking of combinations, do oral agents react with other drugs?**

A In some cases. Any drug or medication has the potential to interact with another substance. Cortisone and other corticosteroids in particular have been known to raise blood-sugar levels and make oral hypoglycaemic agents less effective. Other drugs, stated by British manufacturers to be capable of interactions, are:

- sulphonamides
- aspirin
- phenylbutazone
- cyclophosphamide
- rifampicin
- monoamine oxidase inhibitors (MAOIs)
- diuretics
- oral contraceptives
- bezafibrate
- clofibrate
- oral anticoagulants
- chloramphenicol
- glucagon.

Note that aspirin and some other commonly taken drugs are included in the above list. When in doubt about interactions, even with non-prescription medicines, you should always consult your doctor.

Q   **I've been told not to take oral hypoglycaemics during illness. Why?**

A   It's not that you can't take them, it's that oral therapy may not work. That's because periods of physical stress often create a dramatic jump in blood glucose.

Q   **What do you mean by 'physical stress'?**

A   Those times when you have a fever, cold or flu; when you have a sinus infection or a urinary-tract infection; when you've been injured; or when you are undergoing surgery. During these times, people with type-II diabetes will generally need insulin (usually a human insulin) instead of oral hypoglycaemics. For some people this insulin use is temporary. After the illness has passed, they may go back to oral therapy, again monitoring blood sugar frequently at the start.

Q   **I've read that sometimes, out of the blue, an oral hypoglycaemic stops working. Is that so? Does oral therapy fail?**

A   Yes. Useful as this therapy is for type-II diabetes, about half of the people who use it eventually stop after 5 or 6 years, simply because the drugs no longer work. The failure may be due to an infection, surgery or severe injury, in which case the patient may once again have good luck with the drug after the ailment or injury is cleared up. In other cases, blood-glucose levels become elevated, out of the blue, and the doctor has to increase the dose or prescribe a different agent. No one is quite sure what causes secondary failure, although doctors say it can happen when someone stops exercising or neglects his or her eating plan.

Each year, approximately 5 to 10 per cent of patients on oral therapy experience failure. The medical world hoped that the more recent sulphonylureas would be less vulnerable to this problem, but that doesn't seem to be the case, although results are still coming in on these new drugs. Overall, oral agents fail to bring blood sugar under control in 30 to 40 per cent of people with type-II diabetes.

Q **So, what happens when oral hypoglycaemics fail?**
A For some individuals, insulin is the next step.

INSULIN THERAPY

Q **Insulin? But I thought only people with type-I diabetes used this?**
A Not so. Insulin is used when other therapies have failed. And we must acknowledge that many diabetes therapies do fail. If the object is to achieve normal blood-sugar levels in type-II diabetes, then the medical profession has a fairly poor track record. Only a fraction of patients do well on diet therapy alone, and the primary failure rate of treatment with an oral hypoglycaemic agent may be as high as 30 per cent. This means that, eventually, two thirds of patients with type-II diabetes who are being treated as well as possible, will need insulin.

Injected insulin helps with type-II diabetes because it

gives beta cells in the pancreas a rest – after all, the disease has been forcing them to work overtime. After a period of time, when blood sugar has been controlled, the patient may possibly be able to resume the use of oral agents.

Q **Are there any drawbacks to giving insulin to patients with type-II diabetes?**

A A few. The first is hyperinsulinaemia, which we mentioned before. Giving insulin to insulin-resistant type-II patients may contribute to or exacerbate hyperinsulinaemia, which may be a risk factor for cardiovascular disease. Another area of concern with insulin therapy is its effectiveness in very overweight people. Some extremely obese type-II patients require huge amounts of insulin, and even with large doses they aren't able to control their blood sugar. In addition, insulin tends to promote weight gain, a particularly undesirable effect for type-II patients, as most of them are overweight to begin with.

Q **Are these problems common?**

A Not really. Most people with type-II diabetes do well with insulin.

Q **What will I have to do with the insulin?**

A We recommend that you refer back to Chapter 2 of this book, which reviews the details of insulin injection. Most people with type-II diabetes need to take 2 injections of insulin a day, just like their type-I peers. Many do well taking a mixture of soluble (short-acting insulin) and NPH (intermediate-acting insulin) twice a day – often before breakfast and dinner – which is, again, similar to the most common regimen used by people with type-I diabetes.

Anyone – type-I or type-II – using insulin must monitor blood-glucose levels several times a day. The data derived from these blood-glucose readings provide the doctor and patient with the information needed to make adjustments in insulin doses and to watch for instances of hypoglycaemia – a common problem with insulin use.

NEW THERAPIES

Q **Are doctors developing any new therapies for type-II diabetes?**

A The newest brainchild, called **combination therapy**, is now in clinical trials. It combines oral hypoglycaemic pills with 1 injection of insulin a day, usually a small amount of NPH late in the evening.

Many specialists see great potential in combination therapy, particularly for what they term 'poorly controlled patients'. One of the benefits of this therapy is that less insulin might be used. Indeed, a Finnish study found that type-II patients treated with insulin and sulphonylurea required 50 per cent less insulin compared with an insulin-only group.

As well as the sulphonylureas, the biguanide drug

metformin is also being explored in combination therapy. The good thing about metformin is that it doesn't produce hyperinsulinaemia. All other diabetes therapies produce some degree of hyperinsulinaemia, which increasingly seems related to cardiovascular disease. Considering that 77 per cent of all hospitalizations for diabetes, other than for hypoglycaemia, involve cardiovascular complications, and that 80 per cent of the deaths are cardiac in nature, it's easy to see why doctors are excited about this potential therapy.

Most investigators expect diabetes therapy increasingly to involve combination therapies. However, it may be years before they are available to the average person with diabetes.

Q **Are there any surgical approaches to treating type-II diabetes?**

A Doctors are debating the role of pancreas transplants, beta cell transplants, and/or use of an artificial pancreas for type-II diabetes – the same sort of surgical approaches to type-I diabetes now in clinical investigation and which are discussed in Chapter 2. But these are not options for type-II diabetes at the moment, although they may be in future. The best tools for handling the disease still remain the most fundamental ones: diet and exercise.

Q **So it ultimately all comes back to diet?**

A Absolutely. There is no reason why more people shouldn't succeed in maintaining target blood-sugar levels through a combination of weight loss, careful eating and exercise. It all begins with commitment, willpower and the realization that you, the person with diabetes, have control over your health and your future.

Remember, one-fifth of everyone with type-II diabetes has succeeded in controlling blood sugar through diet.

Q   **Is their diabetes gone forever?**

A   Not really, but as long as they maintain a healthy weight and stick to their eating plan, their blood-glucose levels stay normal, although their blood-sugar levels may creep up every once in a while.

For many people, shedding pounds enables them to wave goodbye to diabetes and to its many related conditions, such as high blood pressure and cardio-vascular disease. Diabetic complications are the subject of our next chapter.

CHAPTER FOUR

DIABETIC COMPLICATIONS

Q **Why do most people with diabetes experience complications?**

A Diabetes has widespread impact, reaching into every corner of the body and touching every system. Its effects are cumulative. The longer someone has diabetes, the greater the risk of experiencing a complication, particularly those affecting the most vulnerable areas: the eyes, the heart, the blood vessels and the feet.

There was a time not so long ago when diabetes was devastating. Many people with diabetes died young; the few who managed to survive were crippled by one or another of the disease's major complications. Then insulin was discovered in 1921, and people with diabetes had a tool to help keep the more debilitating complications in check. Today we know that through careful lifestyle choices, people can delay the onset of diabetic complications and slow the progression of the disease and its related ailments.

Despite these inroads, diabetic complications remain a reality for some people. And in this lies a certain irony:

medical science now helps people with diabetes live longer, but the longer they have the disease, the greater the risk of experiencing any of a variety of related conditions.

Q   **What sorts of conditions are you talking about?**
A   Eye problems, for a start. Diabetes is the major cause of blindness in adults: blindness is five times more prevalent among people with diabetes than among people with normal blood-sugar levels. This blindness is caused by bleeding inside the eyes.

Infections and ulcers in the lower legs and feet are other diabetes-related problems. Arterial obstruction leading to loss of blood supply and gangrene is another major problem. Diabetes is responsible for half of the amputations performed. In addition, diabetes is thought to cause a quarter of kidney failures. And people with diabetes experience heart attacks or strokes twice as often as people who do not have diabetes.

Q   **How can I tell if complications are developing?**
A   Generally, you can't, at least not without undergoing a test or medical examination in a doctor's or specialist's surgery. Diabetes proceeds unnoticed, silently ravaging the body. People with diabetes are often without symptoms until some damage is already done.

There is, however, one sure-fire indication that problems are developing, albeit quietly: persistently high blood-sugar levels. In fact, you might argue (as many doctors do) that high sugar levels are the cause of the problems. It's a message that you've heard before in this book and that you'll hear again: control of blood sugar is all-important.

Q **What is considered a dangerously high blood-sugar level?**

A Today's diabetes experts believe that repeated readings above 13.3 mmol/L (240 mg/dl) are unacceptable. The ideal level is the target set by you and your doctor. It will probably be in the 4.4 to 6.6 mmol/L (80 to 120 mg/dl) range.

Q **Who is more likely to experience complications, someone with type-I diabetes or someone with type-II?**

A Because people with type-I diabetes usually get the disease earlier in life than those with type-II, they have the dubious distinction of running a greater risk of developing complications. For the most part, complications appear in people who have had diabetes for 15 years or more, although certain short-term complications can appear (and disappear) at any time.

Evidence of diabetes-related eye problems, for example, is present after 5 years in 1 per cent of type-I cases; by 14 years this percentage is close to 100.

Once complications begin, they proceed at vastly different rates. The thing to remember is this: every person is different. No one can predict where or when or even if complications will arise. You may never experience problems. But since no one can be certain, it's important to practise sound health habits.

Q **Do all people with diabetes develop these problems?**

A Individuals with type-I tend to develop different problems from those with type-II. For instance, type-I diabetes tends to produce vision problems sooner than type-II diabetes, while type-II diabetes appears to be linked to more heart attacks and strokes.

Q **Will an individual with diabetes develop all these complications?**

A It's entirely possible to experience several types of problems – vision and feet problems, for example. But it's rare indeed to see all diabetic complications in one person.

Q **Is there any way to prevent these problems?**

A Experts believe that good control of diabetes, beginning from the first day diabetes is diagnosed, may prevent many of the common diabetes complications and lessen the severity of other complications. In fact, many people who begin a regimen of blood-sugar control can reverse some of the temporary damage that certain complications cause.

Q **You've mentioned eye problems, blindness, amputation, kidney disease – just how many kinds of diabetes complications are there?**

A Somewhere in the neighbourhood of three dozen, if you count various small conditions and infections. It may be more helpful, however, to look at these problems as falling into two groups.

Diabetes complications are classified as short term (those that strike quickly at any time) and long term (those that develop only after someone has had diabetes for years). The medical profession uses the term **acute** when talking of short-term, rapidly occurring complications, and **chronic** when referring to long-term complications.

Let's look at some of the major problems in both groups.

SHORT-TERM COMPLICATIONS

Q **Are short-term complications less serious than long-term ones?**

A Not necessarily. Short-term complications can occur at any time and can certainly be dangerous – sometimes fatal. But the plus side of short-term problems (if you can think of problems as being positive!) is that they generally can be prevented or reversed. The most common are hypoglycaemia and diabetic ketoacidosis or coma.

HYPOGLYCAEMIA

Q **Hypoglycaemia – you've mentioned this complication before. It's a dangerously low level of blood sugar, right?**

A Right. Usually indicated by blood-glucose readings of

3.4 mmol/L (60 mg/dl) or lower, hypoglycaemia is one of the most common complications of diabetes. People often call this an insulin reaction, but this can be misleading, as you will appreciate once you understand the inter-relationship of insulin dosage (sugar down), food intake (sugar up), diet (sugar down) and exertion (sugar down). Other factors can also influence blood-sugar levels, as we have seen.

The hypoglycaemic attack begins abruptly. Once the cycle of low blood sugar gets under way, it can proceed rapidly. In a matter of hours the person may go from feeling uncomfortable to becoming irritable, perhaps irrational and incoherent. The latter are signals that the brain is no longer getting enough glucose. A person may appear to be drunk. Eventually, if the low sugar levels continue, the person may pass out and go into a coma. Left untreated, hypoglycaemia can cause death.

Doctors sometimes call hypoglycaemia an **iatrogenic** condition, meaning that it can be caused by the *treatment* of the disease.

Q **How can treatment cause this condition?**

A Consider the situation of someone with untreated diabetes: the blood-sugar level is always above normal, so there is no risk of hypoglycaemia, or low blood sugar. Once someone begins to treat his or her diabetes – in other words, using diet, exercise, insulin or medications (oral agents) to maintain blood sugar at normal or near-normal levels – then the risk arises of instances when he or she overshoots the mark, so to speak, and brings the blood sugar down too far.

Q **Who gets insulin reactions?**

A Insulin reactions frequently happen to people who use insulin or oral hypoglycaemic agents, and it's especially prevalent in those people with type-I diabetes who follow a regimen of tight blood-glucose control. (See the discussion of tight control in Chapter 2 for more details.) Achieving a normal blood-sugar level is a delicate balance between sugar and insulin. Too much insulin, relative to the other factors, can send the blood sugar too far down. To be very specific, someone might take too much insulin or too large a dose of an oral hypoglycaemic agent. If the overdose is not counterbalanced by an increased intake of sugar, very low blood-sugar levels may develop.

There are, of course, other ways that someone taking insulin or oral agents might inadvertently cause blood-sugar levels to fall too far.

Q **Such as?**

A Delaying or skipping a meal, not eating enough carbohydrates in a meal, and exercising relatively too much, unexpectedly or at the wrong time of day. Drinking a large quantity of alcohol can sometimes throw blood-sugar levels out of balance.

Q **What are the signs of hypoglycaemia?**

A Early symptoms of hypoglycaemia include:

- weakness
- trembling
- intense hunger
- cold and clammy skin
- sweating
- quick pulse
- headache
- anxiety
- irritability.

Later symptoms include:

- headaches
- confusion
- drowsiness
- unconsciousness
- seizures
- coma.

Affected people who recognize what is happening can put things right by taking sugar. Unfortunately, as we shall see, hypoglycaemia can affect judgement and can prevent the sufferer from realizing what is going on. Treating severe hypoglycaemic reactions requires assistance from another person, as the affected person can no longer help him- or herself.

These may sound fairly clear-cut symptoms, and for most people they serve sufficient warning. Unfortunately, many people experience a situation called **reaction denial**.

Q   **Is this when someone refuses to admit to having an insulin reaction?**

A   Yes, usually because he or she can no longer think clearly because blood-glucose levels in the brain are too low – sometimes 1.1 or 1.7 mmol/L (20 or 30 mg/dl). In such cases a friend or family member must insist that the victim drink something sugary, or eat sugary sweets, to get sugar levels up. After the insulin reaction is over, the person often looks back and says, 'Yes, you were right. I did need more sugar.'

There's a similar problem which isn't exactly reaction denial. It's sometimes referred to as **hypoglycaemic unawareness**.

Q   **What's that?**

A   It's when people *don't experience* the warning signals. Those people with type-I diabetes who follow a tight-control regimen are most likely to have this problem. One team of Australian researchers studied 50 such individuals and found that they couldn't detect the warning signs of hypoglycaemia 64 per cent of the time when using human insulin and 69 per cent of the time when using pork-derived insulin.

Q   **Why don't those people experience any warning signals?**

A   We've come across two explanations. The first attributes it to the fact that when someone maintains blood sugar at near-normal levels, a drop from, say, 4.7 to 3.3 mmol/L (85 mg/dl to 60 mg/dl) is not very dramatic and therefore less noticeable than, say, a drop from 13.3 to 3.3 mmol/L (240 mg/dl to 60 mg/dl) which a person with unstable diabetes might experience.

Researchers offer a more technical explanation: the absence of a hormone called **glucagon**.

Q **What is glucagon?**

A It's a naturally occurring substance, also produced by the pancreas, and found in the blood. It is one of several so-called counter-regulatory hormones that help keep the body's sugar and insulin levels on an even keel. Glucagon is secreted by the pancreas to raise blood-sugar levels when those levels get too low.

In recent years scientists have found that most people with type-1 diabetes gradually lose the ability to produce glucagon in response to low blood-sugar levels. This problem seems to develop during the first 5 years of the disease. Without this 'glucagon response' to low blood sugar, people with diabetes are at great risk of severe hypoglycaemic reactions, particularly with a tight-control insulin regimen. These people often display hypoglycaemic unawareness, because they no longer experience anxiety, shaking or other warning signals. Glucagon can be given by injection to treat a hypoglycaemic attack (see below).

Q **If hypoglycaemia can cause reaction denial and hypoglycaemic unawareness, then how am I to know if I have hypoglycaemia?**

A There's only one certain way to find out: take a

blood-glucose reading. Using a home blood-glucose-measurement kit, and following the guidelines for self-monitoring of blood glucose (BGM), you can get the real facts on the state of your sugar levels. Readings from the kit's blood-glucose meter can disclose what your mood or symptoms may not.

Q **What should be done when blood-sugar levels go down?**

A Many doctors recommend that people with diabetes eat something with carbohydrates when sugar levels get down to 3.3 or 3.8 mmol/L (60 or 70 mg/dl). Below 3.3 mmol/L (60 mg/dl), they should treat the situation like a medical emergency – because it could well be. Again, the first step is to eat or drink something. Traditional recommendations include drinking a small glass of fruit juice or ordinary soft drink (one with sugar), or eating dried fruit, six or seven boiled sweets, two tablespoons of raisins, six jelly beans or several glucose tablets. Once the reaction is treated and the symptoms subside, the person may need to eat an additional small meal or snack to prevent blood sugar from dropping again later in the day.

Your GP can give you additional guidelines for treating insulin reactions, including a list of foods to keep near at hand. It's essential for anyone prone to hypoglycaemia to carry a small amount of sugary foods, such as glucose tablets, sugar lumps or sweets, to be eaten in the event of an insulin reaction.

Q   Let's say the person doesn't get blood-sugar levels up soon enough. What's the next step?

A   At this point, he or she may be disorientated, confused or even unconscious. Since you can't give food or drink by mouth to someone who is unconscious (the person may choke to death), someone will have to inject glucagon. That person might be a family member, a co-worker, friend or flatmate.

Q   Glucagon? Isn't that one of the hormones you talked about earlier?

A   Like the hormone insulin, glucagon is manufactured by pharmaceutical companies for use by people with diabetes and, again like insulin, it is injected with a syringe and needle. A glucagon injection is the way to treat a person who is unconscious because of hypo-glycaemia.

Q   How can I prevent insulin reactions?

A   You can monitor your blood-sugar levels frequently and act accordingly. But it's almost impossible to go through life with diabetes and not experience several insulin reactions. The key is to set up a system that can help you recognize this short-term complication at once and to deal with it quickly and effectively when it does happen.

KETOACIDOSIS

Q   What is this complication, and what causes it?

A   Ketoacidosis, the state that underlies diabetic coma,

primarily affects people with type-I diabetes. There is another form of diabetic coma experienced with type-II diabetes, and we'll discuss that in a moment. Ketoacidosis is caused by a persistently high level of blood sugar, or hyperglycaemia.

Certain situations enable hyperglycaemia to occur:

- too much food
- not enough exercise
- not enough insulin or medication
- physical stress, such as an infection, the flu or another illness
- psychological stress.

Q **A coma is dangerous, I presume?**

A Absolutely. Before insulin was discovered, ketoacidosis was a leading cause of death in people with diabetes. Even today, people who do not control their diabetes can die from diabetic coma. However, most people learn to recognize and treat the early stages of this complication, thus avoiding a tragic outcome.

Q **Does ketoacidosis occur quickly?**

A No, it usually comes on slowly, over the course of many days. The situation develops like this: blood sugar builds up when your cells cannot absorb glucose for use as energy. At this point, the body begins to burn fat as fuel, producing acidic waste products known as ketones. These ketones accumulate in the blood (a situation known as **ketosis**) and eventually work their way into the urine (a situation known as **ketonuria**).

As ketones continue to build up, a tremendous amount of fluid is discharged from the body in the form of urine, and dehydration begins. The blood eventually becomes extremely acidic. At this point, ketoacidosis has set in. If untreated, ketoacidosis affects brain function, leading to loss of consciousness and death.

It may take 12 hours, it may take 36, but ketoacidosis will occur if the person doesn't recognize the symptoms and take steps to lower blood-glucose levels.

Q   **What are the symptoms of ketoacidosis?**

A   The symptoms may include frequent urination and great thirst, fever, vomiting or nausea, blurred vision, abdominal pain, disorientation and drowsiness. Frequent urination, in particular, causes dehydration, which increases the blood acidity caused by the acid ketones. Unconsciousness finally results.

Q   **How can someone with diabetes tell if ketoacidosis is developing?**

A   When the person notices symptoms that resemble those of ketoacidosis, the first step is to check the blood-sugar levels. If those levels are over 13.3 mmol/L (240 mg/dl) for two consecutive tests, the next step is to test the urine for the presence of ketones. Ketones are sometimes referred to as **acetones**, and the urine test for ketones is sometimes called a urine acetone test.

If both blood-sugar and ketone levels are high, the

person should inject a dose of soluble, fast-acting insulin immediately and call the doctor for additional instruction. In most cases, additional insulin doses and exercise can terminate this condition before it reaches the advanced stage – when ketoacidosis must be treated in hospital.

Q **Why is that?**

A Because ketoacidosis is accompanied by dehydration, special care is needed to replace body fluids and treat the body for shock. GPs can monitor blood glucose and other blood chemicals much more easily in a hospital setting, giving additional doses of insulin to the patient when needed. Minerals such as potassium are often very low and must be replaced gradually. When the person's blood chemistry returns to normal, he or she can resume the normal self-care regimen.

Q **At what point does the patient go into a coma?**

A Actually, the term *diabetic coma* is not the same as ketoacidosis. To assume that they are is misleading. You will not be unconscious just because you have a minor degree of ketoacidosis; it's only when the level of ketones rises above a certain point that coma occurs. Obviously, it's not a good idea to let it get to that stage. Any of the symptoms plus ketones in the urine are signals to take immediate action. You can avoid a coma and even hospitalization by acting quickly and taking insulin when blood-sugar levels are high.

Q   You said earlier that people with type-II diabetes may
     experience a different form of coma. What's that?

A   It's known as the **hyperosmolar** or **nonketotic coma**.
     Let's look at it now.

HYPEROSMOLAR, OR NONKETOTIC COMA

Q   How is this different from ketoacidosis, the so-called
     diabetic coma?

A   This is a form of diabetic coma generally experienced by
     people with type-II diabetes. We should note here that
     some people don't distinguish between ketoacidosis
     and hyperosmolar comas, because the symptoms are
     similar and both feature high sugar levels. However, the
     hyperosmolar coma has a different chemical basis.

Q   Could you explain this in simple terms?

A   Basically, in a hyperosmolar coma, ketones do not
     develop as they do in a diabetic coma. As insulin is
     present in the person with type-II diabetes, even though
     it cannot work properly, it prevents the body from
     burning fat as an alternative fuel. If fat isn't burned, then
     ketones aren't produced. Thus the chemical difference
     between ketoacidosis and the hyperosmolar coma:
     Hyperosmolar simply means that too much stuff is
     dissolved in the blood so that the solution is too
     concentrated.

Q   **So it is the high sugar level that causes the coma?**

A   Yes. In a person who is insulin resistant, the body tries to lower blood-glucose levels through the kidneys, which causes the kidneys to work overtime and also causes frequent urination. A tremendous amount of fluid may be lost, causing dehydration and thickening of the blood. Although the blood doesn't become acidic, as in the case of ketoacidosis, it becomes concentrated, which is just as dangerous. Blood concentration due to dehydration is called *hyperosmolar*, which means 'increased concentration of substances in the blood'.

Q   **You said the symptoms are similar to those of ketoacidosis?**

A   This is true in general: frequent urination and great thirst, nausea, abdominal pain, dry skin, disorientation and, later, laboured breathing and drowsiness. Ketones aren't an issue – thus the name nonketotic coma. However, like ketoacidosis, it is a matter of degree before actual coma develops – although the person will probably be disorientated and confused. Indeed, unlike in ketoacidosis, frank coma is not a principal feature of hyperosmolarity unless the affected person develops convulsions. So the name is really misleading. The thing to remember is that very high blood sugar in type-I diabetes means the production of acidic products – ketones – which are very toxic to the brain. Very high blood sugar in type-II diabetes will probably not feature ketones and the effect on the brain is less severe. It is, none the less, quite dangerous.

Q And how do I treat this problem?

A Again, it's important to test your blood-glucose levels regularly. If they are unusually high for several tests in a row, an insulin injection or more diabetes medication and exercise may be called for. A person needs immediate medical assistance when the blood sugar remains over about 22 mmol/L (400 mg/dl) for 12 consecutive hours despite additional doses of insulin. Once dehydration sets in, he or she may have to be hospitalized so that liquids, sugars and other blood chemicals can be stabilized.

Q We've looked at insulin reactions caused by very low blood sugar, and diabetic comas featuring very high blood sugar. How can I tell these two conditions apart?

A In the early phases of each there are differences. In general, an insulin reaction, or low blood sugar, tends to appear abruptly. The person is sweaty, with moist, clammy skin, and is nervous and edgy. Diabetic comas, on the other hand, develop over a period of days. Someone with an impending coma will have dry skin, feel nauseated and be drowsy or dazed.

The thing to remember is that each person has different responses to high and low sugar and to ketoacidosis. As someone with diabetes, it's wise to know what your responses tend to be. Use self-monitoring of blood glucose to track your sugar patterns and guard against these short-term but potentially deadly complications.

LONG-TERM COMPLICATIONS

Q **How do long-term complications differ from short-term ones?**

A Long-term, chronic complications take more time to develop, and once they arrive are usually permanent, or at least less likely to disappear. Many long-term complications are related to those structures that distribute blood throughout the body: the small and large blood vessels, or arteries. Although scientists are not certain how it happens, they think that years of carrying blood with high sugar levels eventually damages or impairs blood vessels. The faulty metabolism of someone with diabetes may also create some chemical change that makes blood vessels more vulnerable to damage. Either way, many diabetic complications are **vascular** complications – that is, pertaining to arteries.

EYE PROBLEMS

Q **What kind of eye problems does diabetes cause?**

A They include minor problems in focusing, premature development of **cataracts** and various degrees of retinal damage (otherwise known as diabetic retinopathy).

Q **How common are these problems?**

A It's very likely that someone with diabetes will experience at least one of these problems in the course of his or her lifetime. Most people who have had diabetes for

5 to 10 years show some signs of eye damage, although it may only be slight.

Q **What about focusing problems?**

A These are transient and occur when the blood-sugar levels are very high. They are due to changes in the curvature and size of the internal lenses of the eyes as a result of temporary variations in the amount of water in the lenses. This occurs as an effect of what is called osmotic pressure – the force that causes fluid to flow through body membranes from areas of high concentration of dissolved substances to areas of low concentration. Temporary short sight caused in this way will correct itself when the blood-sugar levels are put right.

Q **I've heard about cataracts. They are a clouding of the internal lens in the eye, right?**

A Right. They don't affect the corneas, just the tiny inner lenses that lie behind the pupils. Diabetes can cause two kinds of cataract. Rarely, it may cause an acute onset of cataract in young people. Such cataracts come on rapidly and affect both eyes severely so that the person concerned moves from normal visions to blindness in a few days. In most cases of juvenile-onset diabetes, however, cataract is not a problem. You will understand that cataracts are a very common problem in older people, including those who don't have diabetes. However, the evidence suggests that diabetes accelerates cataract development, which is one reason that people with diabetes generally develop cataracts sooner than people who do not have diabetes. What seems to happen is that ordinary old-age-related cataracts occur rather earlier in people with diabetes than in those without it.

Q **What makes this happen?**
A It's all part of that intricate and still incompletely under-stood relationship between high blood-sugar levels and tissue damage. One theory proposes that when people have had diabetes for an extended period of time, sugar by-products begin to build up in the lens of the eye, eventually leading to cataracts.

Q **How are cataracts treated?**
A Mild lens opacities are not too disabling and are often left as they are – but an individual with diabetes is encouraged to work at keeping blood-sugar levels within the normal range, which seems to slow the progression of complications.

Once severe opacities develop, however, ophthal-mologists believe that the best course of action is to remove the affected lenses and replace them with an artificial lens in each eye, also known as an **intraocular lens**. This operation can be done by day care surgery and the results are excellent.

Although cataracts certainly impede sight, they are much less troublesome than another long-term compli-cation, diabetic retinopathy.

Q **What is retinopathy?**

A It is damage to or disease of the retina, the delicate membrane that lines the inside wall of the back and sides of the eye. The retina responds to light and receives the image formed by the lens system.

Q **What causes diabetic retinopathy?**

A In general, changes or abnormalities in the small blood vessels of the retina – changes that take years to occur.

Q **Is retinopathy common?**

A Yes. Some degree is present in almost all people with long-standing diabetes. Diabetic retinopathy is the most frequent cause of severe vision loss in people 20 to 74 years old. Fortunately, early diagnosis and prompt treatment can often prevent blindness.

Q **Who gets retinopathy?**

A Almost everyone with diabetes develops this complication, but the first to feel its impact are people with type-I, who frequently develop a mild form of this condition within 5 years of diagnosis of diabetes. In fact, there's a strong correlation between the amount of time someone has had diabetes and the development of retinopathy.

Q **Correlation? What do you mean by that?**

A Quite simply, the longer you have diabetes, the greater your chance of developing significant retinopathy. Within 10 years of diabetes diagnosis, half of all people with type-I diabetes and a quarter with type-II have some damage to their retinas. By 20 years after the onset of diabetes, nearly everyone with type-I diabetes and over 60 per cent with type-II have some degree of retinopathy.

Q **How dangerous is this complication?**
A Retinopathy is not something to take lightly. Among those with type-I diabetes, retinopathy is responsible for four-fifths of all cases of blindness; among those with type-II, the number is one-third. Of course, not all cases of retinopathy result in blindness. The condition ranges in severity from mild to advanced.

Q **You mentioned that some people develop a mild form of retinopathy. Are you saying that there's more than one form of this disease?**
A The medical profession describes two forms of diabetic retinopathy: **background retinopathy** and **proliferative retinopathy**.

Q **What is background retinopathy?**
A This mild, early form of retinopathy is characterized by gradual narrowing or weakening of the small blood vessels in the eye. Small bulges (called **microaneurysms**) develop on the smallest vessels. Eventually a few tiny vessels, here and there, may tear or break and bleed (known in medical parlance as a **haemorrhage**), leaving small flame-shaped red blotches on the retina.

   Most people with diabetes develop background

retinopathy, but in most cases the condition remains at a mild level. Vision is not affected unless blood vessels break and leak fluid into the **macula**, an area of the retina responsible for sharp, fine vision – the kind of vision you need to read this book. When fluid leaks into the macula, it swells and damages the function of this important part of the retina. This situation is called a **macular oedema**, and it leads to blurred vision.

Q **Can a macular oedema be treated?**

A The swelling is sometimes treated in patients who appear to be at high risk of blindness with a high-tech procedure known as **photocoagulation**. This is when a precise laser beam is used to sear shut the leaking blood vessels. This kind of photocoagulation doesn't cure retinopathy, but it can delay the loss of vision by a number of years or, in some cases, stop progression. For the most part, however, because background retinopathy is mild, surgical treatment isn't necessary.

Q **How does proliferative retinopathy differ from background retinopathy?**

A As its name suggests, this severe form of retinopathy develops when a frond-like network of new, fragile blood vessels proliferate in the retina at the site of previous breakages or haemorrhages. Over time the new, fragile vessels may tear and bleed into the **vitreous humour**, the clear, gel-like material that fills the centre of the eye. A small leakage of blood won't dim vision, but the major haemorrhages associated with proliferative retinopathy may be large enough to affect sight, in which case they are known as **vitreous haemorrhages**.

As the eye tries to repair the damage caused by these haemorrhages, scar tissue forms in the vitreous. The build-up of scar tissue may eventually pull on and damage the retina, resulting in partial loss of sight, or it may displace or cause the retina to become detached, resulting in total loss of vision.

Q   **Is there any way to tell that either form of retinopathy is developing – before blindness sets in?**

A   For the most part, people can have severe eye damage without knowing it, because the damage may not affect vision and may cause no pain. Eye examinations with a tool called an **ophthalmoscope** are used to detect damage to the retina.

Q   **Is this an examination my GP can do?**

A   Yes, although several studies indicate that doctors who are not **ophthalmologists** are not skilled in detecting either background or proliferative retinopathy, and may find these conditions in only 50 per cent of the people who have them. That's not a particularly encouraging track record, but it has to be acknowledged that using an ophthalmoscope is a difficult skill that requires a lot of practice and experience. Ophthalmologists do not use ophthalmoscopes without first putting in drops to widen the pupils of the eyes, and then they will always work in the dark so as to get maximal contrast. GPs will often try to examine retinas in bright light and without dilating the patient's pupils first. In short, examining retinas to detect diabetic changes is a job for the experts and should be done by an ophthalmologist in an Eye Department. Every patient with diabetes should be referred for such examination.

Of course, there are some obvious indications to the person with diabetes that something has happened to the eye. Partial loss of vision – even if very slight – is an indication of a problem. 'Floaters' and 'cobwebs' are terms that people have used to describe vision problems caused by tiny haemorrhages in the eye. A sudden, painful loss of vision may indicate a major haemorrhage. Naturally, it's best to detect retinopathy before it reaches this stage.

Q **Can anything be done for retinopathy once it reaches the advanced stage?**

A Yes: photocoagulation – the use of intensely bright focused light or laser beams – not to seal leaking retinal blood vessels or reattach a detached retina, but to destroy as much as possible of the peripheral (and un-needed) parts of the retina, so as to reduce the overall metabolic requirements of this part of the eye. This apparently destructive process is called pan-photocoagulation and it has been found to be a valuable way of preventing the growth of the new and fragile blood vessels from which vitreous haemorrhages occur. In some people, pan-photocoagulation is enough to stop the progression of diabetic retinopathy.

Vitrectomy is another, more intricate surgical procedure used in people with proliferative retinopathy. In this procedure, a doctor removes the vitreous to clear out the light-blocking haemorrhage, uses micro-surgery to repair the retina, if necessary, and then replaces the vitreous with a saline solution.

Q How effective are these eye operations?

A Photocoagulation and vitrectomy prevent deterioration of vision in around 60 per cent of patients. For instance, laser therapy reportedly reduces the rate of vision loss by 50 per cent in people with proliferative retinopathy and macular oedema, conditions which often exhibit no symptoms. Vitrectomy reportedly improves visual acuity to 6/12 or better in 36 per cent of treated eyes. That's the good news.

Q You mean to say there's bad news?

A Well, as you know, no surgery is free of potential complications. With vitrectomy, for example, the overall complication rate is about 25 per cent.

Q What about taking a different tack – are there any nonsurgical techniques available to treat retinopathy?

A Medical research is looking at ways of slowing or even preventing the progression of retinopathy.

Several studies have shown that people with type-I diabetes who maintain near-normal levels of blood sugar over a long period of time – at least 7 years – are significantly less likely to develop severe retinopathy.

These patients followed a tight-control regimen, using either continuous subcutaneous infusion pumps or multiple insulin injections. (*See the discussion of tight control in Chapter 2 for a refresher in what this therapy entails.*)

Q **Is there anything else that might prevent eye damage?**

A Scientists are hoping to discover why high levels of blood glucose damage the body's blood vessels. One theory is that an enzyme called an **aldose reductase**, which converts glucose into a sugar alcohol called **sorbitol**, may play a role in triggering diabetes complications. For that reason, researchers are looking into a class of drugs called **aldose reductase inhibitors**, which block the actions of the enzyme. They hope these drugs can reduce the chance of developing retinopathy and other long-term complications. Clinical trials are under way.

Although these new treatments sound promising, the key action in the here and now is proper eye examination by an expert and getting prompt ophthalmic care for retinopathy, particularly if you have macular oedema or proliferative retinopathy.

Q **Why is that?**

A Research has shown that there is a 16 per cent risk of severe vision loss if proliferative retinopathy is left untreated for 2 years. That may sound a small risk, but is it worth taking? You and your doctor must decide.

Q I've heard that pregnant women with diabetes are more likely to develop retinopathy. Is that true?

A A woman with type-I, type-II or gestational diabetes who has no retinopathy before pregnancy is unlikely to develop retinopathy during pregnancy. However, the story is different for women with diabetes who already have some retinal damage when they become pregnant. About 5 to 12 per cent of women with diabetes with mild retinopathy will suffer worsening of their retinopathy. Women with diabetes who already have moderate to severe retinopathy are at greater risk during pregnancy. In recent studies, about 47 per cent of pregnant women with diabetes had an increase in severity in retinal damage, and 5 per cent developed proliferative retinopathy.

Q What causes these rapid changes?

A They may be due to the increased levels of hormones that accompany pregnancy. Pregnancy-induced or chronic high blood pressure is thought to play a role, too. In one study, 55 per cent of pregnant women with diabetes who had high blood pressure in addition to retinopathy had worsening of their retinopathy, compared with 25 per cent of the women who had normal blood pressure.

Q Let's say a pregnant woman already has some sign of retinal damage. Would lowering blood-pressure levels slow the progression of retinopathy?

A Probably, say the experts. Doctors have also found that treating a woman's retinopathy with photocoagulation can help reduce the risk of progression *if* the laser treatment is done before she becomes pregnant.

Like all people with diabetes who have retinopathy, pregnant women should get regular eye examinations to monitor the course and development of this complication.

NEPHROPATHY

Q What is this?

A Officially known as diabetic **nephropathy**, it's a type of kidney disease which can lead to kidney failure. Nephropathy tends to develop in people who have had diabetes for 20 years or more. It used to be that a third of all people with type-I diabetes developed nephropathy, but today's treatment methods and the emphasis on better blood-sugar control are shrinking that percentage. People with type-II diabetes develop nephropathy only infrequently.

Q Why is nephropathy a problem?

A We can answer that by looking first at what the kidneys do.

The kidneys are small organs located at the back near the waist. Inside the kidneys are small blood vessel tufts, called **glomeruli**, which act as filters, removing wastes from the blood and discharging them through the urine. Useful products, such as **protein** and glucose, are not discharged but are retained in the bloodstream.

Nephropathy is the condition in which small arteries in the kidneys become hardened and the glomeruli become damaged (in much the same way that the small vessels of the eye become damaged during retinopathy). The kidneys ultimately fail in their job of filtering out wastes. People with kidney failure must go on **dialysis** (the use of a machine to filter blood) or have a kidney transplant; otherwise, lethal levels of wastes and toxins build up in their bodies.

Q **What causes nephropathy?**

A High blood-sugar levels, for a start. Also, high blood pressure increases the likelihood of kidney complications. Frequent urinary-tract infections add to the problem, because an infection can easily spread to the kidneys and damage them.

Q **How does someone with diabetes find out if kidney damage is developing?**

A Early warning signs are likely to be detected only by urine and blood tests. The possibility must be suspected in anyone with retinopathy of any degree. Retinopathy is an indication that the kind of blood vessel damage that causes nephropathy is occurring. This is another reason for proper eye examination.

Just as the kidneys lose their ability to discharge

wastes, they also lose their ability to retain protein and glucose. Sugar and protein begin to show up in the urine tests in larger and larger amounts. Blood tests detect high levels of urea nitrogen and creatinine, which also indicate kidney damage.

Q **Is there any way to treat kidney problems before kidney failure occurs?**

A The wisest step for all people with diabetes is to have proper and regular medical checks. Urine tests, not just for sugar and ketones, but also for protein and other abnormal constituents, are essential. Blood tests are needed to check kidney function. Occasionally, it may even be necessary for a small sample of kidney tissue to be taken for examination – a kidney biopsy. This is done using a special needle. Such people should also take urinary-tract infections seriously. Talk with a doctor about what to do when they develop. Remember, infections can back up the urinary system and spread to the kidneys, impairing their function.

If signs of developing kidney problems are detected, doctors often emphasize a regimen of tight blood-sugar control and a low-protein diet (see *Chapter 5*) to ease some of the stress on the kidneys. If nephropathy progresses, however, the affected person may ultimately have to undergo kidney dialysis. Kidney transplantation is another option for some.

CARDIOVASCULAR COMPLICATIONS

Q   **What do you mean by 'cardiovascular complications' – and how are they related to diabetes?**

A   The word **cardiovascular** means 'of the heart and blood vessels'. Cardiovascular complications are problems such as angina, heart attack, stroke and others related to reduced supply of blood to parts of the body. Just as diabetes changes the shape of the small blood vessels (known as **microvascular** changes), it also appears to thicken and obstruct the walls of the large blood vessels, thus restricting blood flow. These are called **macrovascular** changes. Macrovascular changes (such as hardening of the arteries) have been called the 'underlying event' behind most cardiovascular disease. There's no doubt about it – cardiovascular complications are very serious side-effects of diabetes.

Q   **Who is at risk of developing heart attacks and strokes?**

A   Just having diabetes increases a person's risk of experiencing a stroke, regardless of whether or not the person has other risk factors.

Q   **What other risk factors exist?**

A   Neglecting exercise, eating a high-fat diet, having high blood pressure and smoking cigarettes – each of these confers more risk. High blood pressure alone is a major cause of strokes.

Q **Are cardiovascular complications more common in men than in women?**

A In the general population, yes: women experience strokes and heart attacks less frequently than men.

Among people with diabetes, however, the answer to that question is no. Men and women with diabetes, particularly with type-II diabetes, suffer equally poor outcomes after heart attacks. They have a higher cardiovascular death rate than people who do not have diabetes, and they are less likely to survive a heart attack than are those who do not have the disease.

Q **That's strange – women generally seem to have a biological advantage. Why does diabetes change this?**

A Diabetes appears to reduce this advantage, at least where heart attacks are concerned. Compared with men who do not have diabetes, men with diabetes have about twice the average risk of developing cardiovascular disease; women with diabetes have three to five times the average risk of developing cardiovascular disease.

Q **Those are very big differences between people with diabetes and those without it. Besides the obvious steps of lowering blood sugar and losing weight, are there any other ways people with diabetes can help prevent heart problems?**

A Cholesterol and **triglycerides** are two other things to focus on if they wish to spare their hearts.

Q   **Why is that?**

A   No doubt you are well aware of the role high cholesterol levels play in heart disease. Cholesterol is a fat-like substance that comes from meat and dairy products and is found in all the body's cells and in the bloodstream. High levels of cholesterol in the blood, or **hypercholesterolaemia**, have been implicated in the development of heart disease in general and the common and serious arterial disease atherosclerosis in particular. It is the atherosclerosis that causes the heart disease.

What you may not know is that people with diabetes tend to have higher blood-cholesterol levels than other people. They also tend to have higher levels of **low-density lipoproteins (LDL)**, what some call the 'bad cholesterol' because it aids in the deposit of fats on artery and cell walls. As if that weren't bad enough, people with diabetes tend to have lower levels of the 'good cholesterol', or **high-density lipoprotein (HDL)**, the substance that escorts excess cholesterol from the body. Both of these facts are likely to promote the development of atherosclerosis. All of this is unpleasant news for the cardiovascular system.

Q   **And those triglycerides you mentioned – what are they?**

A   Triglycerides are the standard form of fat in the body – the kind we all know about and which accumulates in excess because we eat too much. High levels of triglycerides in the blood (**hypertriglyceridaemia**) may not directly cause atherosclerosis, but may accompany other abnormalities which speed its development.

Q **Have people with diabetes got high levels of triglycerides?**

A Yes. Combine high triglyceride levels of 200 to 500 mg/dl with cholesterol levels between 200 and 300 mg/dl, and you have *combined hyperlipidaemia* (meaning altogether too much fat). Triglycerides over 500 mg/dl and/or cholesterol levels over 300 mg/dl are called *massive hyperlipidaemia* – a dangerous state of affairs. Combined and massive hyperlipidaemia are found in over 30 per cent of all people with diabetes – and approximately two to three times more frequently than in people without diabetes.

We'll talk more about cholesterol and triglycerides in the next chapter when we examine diet. For now, it's enough to say that any person with diabetes who improves his or her cholesterol picture can protect against developing cardiovascular problems. Evidence suggests that for every 1 per cent reduction in blood-cholesterol level, there is a 2 per cent reduction in coronary-artery disease.

Q **Is there anything else people with diabetes can do to guard against heart attacks?**

A The medical world has found some benefit in the daily intake of a simple pill – aspirin.

Q **Aspirin? Why is that?**

A A curious thing happened during the course of a clinical study known as the Early Treatment Diabetic Retinopathy Study. This study was designed to gauge the effects of aspirin on diabetic retinopathy, and it included 3,700 people with type-I and type-II diabetes. Half took 2 aspirins a day, the other half took a placebo. It turned out that the aspirin had no effect, positive or negative, on retinopathy. But something positive did come out of it: people taking aspirin were 17 per cent less likely to have a heart attack during the 5 years of the study.

Aspirin can't solve all the cardiovascular woes of someone with diabetes, nor is aspirin useful for everyone. But it would be worth a trip to the doctor to discuss what aspirin can do for you. Remember, however, that aspirin is in the list of drugs that can cause interactions with the oral hypoglycaemic drugs used in type-II diabetes.

NEUROPATHY

Q **What is this?**

A Quite simply, neuropathy is nerve damage. The word *damage* suggests something irrevocable and permanent; actually, this is one long-term complication of diabetes that can appear and disappear in a short period of time. It also varies in intensity, ranging from mild discomfort to severe, disabling pain.

Q **What causes neuropathy?**

A As is true of many diabetes complications, the answer to this question has the medical profession stumped. It's thought that something interferes with the body's nerve pathways so that nerve impulses are no longer transmitted properly. The culprit may be uncontrolled blood-sugar levels (although many people with good control develop this complication), or it may be that the nerves are somehow damaged during the metabolic changes of diabetes.

Q Is it common?

A Yes. It's estimated that some form of nerve damage affects 60 to 70 per cent of people with diabetes at some point in their lives. Some doctors claim that it's often the first noticeable sign of diabetes, particularly in type-II diabetes. Unfortunately, neuropathy mimics many other medical conditions, so it's often initially diagnosed as something else.

The medical profession divides neuropathy into two forms: **peripheral** and **autonomic**.

Q What is peripheral neuropathy?

A The most common form of nerve damage, it's sometimes called *sensory neuropathy* because it often creates odd sensations (or, in some cases, loss of sensation) in the legs, feet and hands.

Q Could you describe those odd sensations?

A They include numbness, tingling, muscle weakness and sporadic shooting pains. These sensations can be mild or they can be annoying. Some people experience double vision for varying periods of time; others have great difficulty walking because of pain or because they lose some control of leg movements. Neuropathy has been known to interfere with sleep or rest.

In general, peripheral neuropathy is a temporary condition – one that disappears as mysteriously as it appears. However, it can lead to injury in cases where the person with diabetes feels no sensations of pain. This often happens on the bottoms of the feet, resulting in some of the foot problems that we'll be discussing shortly.

Q **What is autonomic neuropathy?**

A A less common complication, perhaps experienced by 20 per cent of people with diabetes, autonomic neuropathy is damage of the nerves that control various bodily functions, such as the digestive system, urinary tract and cardiovascular system.

Autonomic neuropathy leads to many inconvenient problems:

- When it affects the nerves around the stomach, bladder and bowels, it can cause vomiting, constipation and feelings of bloatedness.
- When it affects the nerves that control the contraction of blood vessels, a condition called **orthostatic hypotension** may develop. This is a sudden drop in blood pressure when a person gets up after reclining.
- **Impotence**, the loss of the ability to have an erection, is also related to, although not entirely caused by, neuropathic damage.

Q   **Can these problems be treated?**

A   Doctors often prescribe drugs to treat the symptoms of these different problems – for example, to relax muscles if the problem is constipation. Exercise helps some people; others benefit from bed rest. Because neuropathy varies tremendously from person to person, treating it is often a matter of trial and error.

Drugs to treat or prevent nerve damage do not yet exist, although researchers are conducting studies using aldose reductase inhibitors – experimental drugs discussed earlier in relation to retinopathy.

FOOT PROBLEMS

Q   **How does diabetes affect the feet?**

A   Cardiovascular complications damage blood vessels and diminish blood flow to the legs and feet. Add damage to the nerves of the legs and feet through neuropathy and you've laid the groundwork for serious foot ailments.

Q   **How often do these ailments show up?**

A   In about half of people with diabetes for 20 years or more. The plot then proceeds like this: when people with diabetes lose sensation in their lower legs and feet, they are less likely to notice damage to the skin and tissues – problems like cuts, bruises, blisters, bunions, corns, callouses, ingrown toenails or even athlete's foot. Such seemingly minor injuries can progress to an infection known as a neuropathic ulcer.

Q **Wait a minute – a blister can turn into an ulcer? How can that be?**

A Let's say you have a new pair of shoes and one has chafed and rubbed one foot raw. The area is red and inflamed. Once an inflammation or infection begins, its swelling compresses the blood vessels and arteries, which are already damaged or narrowed by diabetes. These factors diminish the flow of blood to the irritated area, meaning that fresh oxygen and infection-fighting blood cells have more difficulty getting to the problem site.

All of this sets the stage for a serious infection. Once infection sets in, it's difficult to treat. Antibiotics, which are carried in the blood, can't reach the infected area efficiently.

Q **Do foot ulcers tend to develop in a certain area?**

A Yes. About 80 per cent of these problems occur on the bottom of feet that have lost sensation. The real danger with the combination of infection and reduced blood flow is **gangrene**. If blood flow were to be completely blocked, the cells served by the obstructed blood vessels would die. Once gangrene sets in, the only safe thing to do is to amputate the dead tissue.

Q **Is amputation common among people with diabetes?**

A According to an article in *Archives of Internal Medicine*, 'It has been estimated that the lifetime risk of a lower-extremity amputation is 5 to 15 per cent among diabetic individuals, a risk 15 times that of the non-diabetic population'.

Many thousands of diabetes-related amputations are performed each year. As is true with all diabetic complications, certain factors increase the risk of ending up with an amputation: being male, being African and having a history of smoking. The risk increases with age, too.

Q   **Is there anyway to find out if a blood vessel is about to become blocked?**

A   Coldness of an extremity, or poor or absent pulses are obvious clinical signs. Blockages in large vessels, such as those of the legs, can be spotted with an x-ray called an **angiogram**. Another useful method is to use a technique called Doppler ultrasound. This can actually measure the rate of blood flow through an artery and indicate whether there is significant loss of flow.

Bypass surgery may be performed to detour blood around the blockage. In this surgery, a piece of a healthy vein is taken from an area of the body (possibly the thigh) that can spare it and is attached at either end of the obstruction. The new vein bypasses the block and directs blood to cells that had been receiving an inadequate supply. It's one way of preventing gangrene.

Q   **Is there any other way to prevent gangrene and amputation?**

A   Amputation doesn't have to happen. With proper foot care, many if not most amputations may well be avoided.

How to care for your feet, how to monitor your blood-sugar levels, how to design and follow a sound eating plan – in short, how to prevent diabetic complications from developing in the first place – are covered in the next chapter. Read on!

CHAPTER FIVE

SELF-CARE: PUTTING
YOURSELF IN CONTROL

Q   **From all that I've learned from this book, diabetes is a complicated disease. Will self-care really make a difference?**

A   Absolutely. Unlike many other illnesses, *the control of diabetes rests in the hands of the patient.* Self-care is not just important, it is absolutely essential.

This chapter, and indeed, this entire book, is designed to help each person with diabetes take charge of his or her own treatment. Keep in mind that the overall goal of any treatment is to control blood sugar – to keep it within normal limits. Achieving that entails re-evaluating your lifestyle, adopting a new meal plan and a regular exercise routine, and making a commitment to self-monitoring of blood glucose. It also entails being aware of the symptoms and dangers of the potential complications of diabetes – those problems discussed in Chapter 4.

Q   **That's a lot of responsibility! Where do I begin?**

A   If you have type-I diabetes, you need to understand the

ways in which insulin, food and exercise affect blood sugar. Insulin has been discussed in depth in Chapter 2; food and exercise are addressed in this chapter.

If you have type-II diabetes, you need to understand the role of obesity, exercise and food consumption in insulin resistance. You may have to lose weight and become more physically active. These latter two things make it easier for your body to produce and use insulin.

Q   **Isn't there any easier way round all this?**

A   Alas, no. The fact of the matter remains: managing your diabetes is demanding and, at times, difficult. It's a daily, lifelong process. But the alternative – neglecting the disease – poses such demonstrable drawbacks that most people opt for self-care.

As we mentioned at the start of this book, the real goal is to control your diabetes, instead of letting it control you. And the encouraging news is that control is literally in your hands!

BLOOD-GLUCOSE MONITORING

Q   **What is blood-glucose monitoring?**

A   We're referring to self-monitoring of blood glucose, or BGM, the hands-on method of tracking blood sugar. With BGM, you can test your blood-sugar level at home, in the office, on the road – anywhere and any time, as often as you wish. It gives people with diabetes a new level of flexibility – they don't have to make a trip to a doctor's surgery whenever they want an accurate blood-glucose reading, as was the case years ago.

Because BGM can provide the information needed to balance food intake, exercise and insulin or medication, it has become the mainstay of diabetes-management plans. Not all doctors are keen on self-care and self-testing, but the medical profession as a whole has embraced self-monitoring of blood glucose, and it is certainly approved of by the official diabetes associations. It may well be the best invention since the discovery of insulin.

Q **How do people with diabetes perform BGM?**

A Using a special needle called a **lancet**, a person pricks his or her finger and then places a drop of blood either on a test strip or on a specially treated sensor pad on a glucose meter (a device about the size of a pocket calculator). Some test strips change colour depending upon the amount of glucose in the blood, and the colour is compared to a master chart. Other strips are inserted into a glucose meter. The blood-glucose meter indicates just how many millimoles of glucose are present in a litre of blood. In the US, the earlier system of units (milligrams of glucose per decilitre of blood) are still used. The reading appears on the meter's display panel in numbers, and the whole test is done within 45 seconds to 2 minutes.

Q **Self-monitoring sounds so simple. What can it achieve?**

A A great deal. Self-monitoring is valuable for anyone who is at all concerned about managing his or her diabetes. Because the process is relatively quick, it can be done many times a day, giving the person a clear picture of how the blood-glucose level fluctuates throughout the day. When blood sugar slides outside the target range, the person can take action.

Q **Should all people with diabetes self-monitor their blood-sugar levels?**

A These days, self-monitoring is recommended for anyone who uses insulin – whether the person has type-I, type-II or gestational diabetes. Many doctors insist that adjustments in insulin doses should be based on blood-glucose measurements. One reason is that even an identical dose of insulin will be absorbed differently from day to day, depending on factors such as insulin sensitivity, exercise, stress, types of food eaten and hormonal changes (puberty, the menstrual cycle, pregnancy).

Self-monitoring is also recommended when someone begins insulin therapy or changes to a new insulin species, brand or dose. (*See Chapter 2 for a review of insulin terms.*) During the adjustment or transition period, the person with diabetes uses BGM to track blood-glucose levels carefully and ensure they are within target ranges.

BGM is also recommended for those people with type-II diabetes who are using oral hypoglycaemic agents, because such people face the danger of very low blood sugar (hypoglycaemia) when using these drugs.

Further, there are additional circumstances in which doctors say BGM is mandatory.

Q   **What are these circumstances?**

A   BGM is required for people who are following a tight-control regimen, whether via insulin pump or frequent insulin injections. As we discussed in Chapters 2 and 4, people following a tight-control regimen are more able to keep their blood-sugar levels on a near-normal, even keel, but they are prone to frequent bouts of hypo-glycaemia, or dangerously low blood sugar. Frequent self-monitoring can flag falling blood-sugar levels before they become disruptive.

Another circumstance which calls for BGM is illness, sometimes referred to as physical stress. Illness wreaks havoc with the body's blood-sugar levels, often increas-ing sugar even if someone does not eat or drink. Thus, people with diabetes generally need to take more insulin when they are sick. But how much more? The results of self-monitoring can guide them and their doctors in making that decision. In fact, in any case where they are forced to stray from their regular medication plans, BGM is essential.

Q   **Do other circumstances call for self-monitoring of blood glucose?**

A   People who have wide swings in blood-sugar levels often turn to BGM to find out why. You may have heard of the term **brittle diabetes**; it describes a rare condition, generally found only among people with type-I diabetes, in which blood-sugar levels fluctuate dramatically from day to day.

Q **What causes brittle diabetes?**

A Wide swings may be caused by poor management of the disease. Or they may have at their root a completely different hormonal disorder, another disease, or the side-effects of drugs. At any rate, self-monitoring can help someone with diabetes track sugar swings and determine how much insulin is necessary, depending upon each day's blood-sugar levels.

As we mentioned earlier, BGM is growing in standing within the medical profession. Your doctor may proffer other reasons to practice this simple self-care technique.

Q **You mentioned that people with diabetes can monitor their sugar levels as often as they want. Is there a required minimum?**

A Frequency is determined by the patient and his or her doctor, although most would agree that haphazard or infrequent measurement – say, only once a week – gives too little information to go on. That said, there are some commonly recommended measurement patterns. For instance, people just beginning BGM may be instructed to check their blood sugar four to eight times a day, including first thing in the morning, before and after each meal, and last thing before bed.

People using insulin (including people with type-I and

type-II diabetes) may average four checks a day: before each meal and late in the evening. People with type-II diabetes who have their sugar under control have the greatest flexibility. Their monitoring schedule might include a morning check four to seven times a week, along with the occasional before-meal or bedtime test.

Q **Am I correct in assuming that people with diabetes generally test their blood before meals?**

A Those who use insulin need these readings to determine how much insulin to take. Some people like to take the occasional reading after a meal (known as a **postprandial** reading), because that's the time when blood sugar shoots up. It can help to gauge how high sugar goes after food consumption.

Q **Are there other times when people with diabetes should monitor their blood sugar?**

A To be precise, there are other times when they should monitor *more frequently* than they usually do – during illness, changes in medication, travel or any change in routine.

Q **Would something like a change in job be included?**

A Yes – basically any change in lifestyle, including a new exercise pattern, a different diet (which may occur when visiting friends or relatives, for example), relocation, job change, marriage, retirement.

Travel through several time zones, especially by air, makes it more difficult to time medications and meals.

Here, BGM can give a person with diabetes the information he or she needs for dose adjustments. Doctors can give special advice about insulin administration when travelling great distances, such as overseas. Self-monitoring will still be important, though. In addition, someone can voluntarily increase the frequency of monitoring whenever he or she wants more information about what's happening in the body.

Q **So BGM is primarily used for adjusting insulin doses?**
A In the short term, self-monitoring tells you what action you need to take to get blood sugar within the target range set by you and your doctor. But BGM is also used to build a larger picture – a month-by-month, year-by-year image of what doctors call **glycaemic control**, or overall control of blood sugar.

BGM enables people with diabetes to build a data base of sorts. Toward this end, many of them plot graphs or start a notebook or diary and record in it the results of their blood-glucose tests. Some of the new blood-glucose meters store this information in an electronic memory. Over time, these details disclose to users how their blood sugar reacts to exercise, to certain foods, to travel and to other environmental factors. With information in hand, people then discuss results with their doctors during routine consultation visits. Ultimately, all of these pieces of information help to fine-tune the diabetes-management programme.

Another benefit of getting to know what's normal for your body is being able to spot a developing problem or emergency, such as an unusually high, or unusually low, blood-glucose reading.

Q If I measure my blood sugar four times a day, won't that get expensive?

A Unfortunately, at the time of writing, meters and finger pricking devices are still not available on the National Health Service. Testing strips can be prescribed, however.

Meters are not particularly expensive, at any rate, and are well worth the price. Among those who use these devices, the cost of meters and supplies may be around £200 a year. Part of this price depends on your choice of equipment.

New versions of blood-glucose kits arrive on the market every season. The trend is toward developing new products that make self-testing simpler, more convenient and quicker. Blood-glucose meters, for example, have become smaller and less cumbersome in recent years – good news if you're inclined to carry a meter along with you on your daily travels.

If you are a private patient, BGM is actually a small part of the total cost of diabetes care. Add in the cost of blood tests performed in your doctor's surgery (we discuss those later in this chapter), and the annual bill for blood monitoring can easily exceed £500 – an amount covered by many (but not all) private health insurers. Yet if self-monitoring delays or prevents the pain, the aggravation and the cost of diabetic complications, then that money is well spent.

Q **Are there any measurement tools besides test strips and glucose meters?**

A A device with a new approach to measuring blood-glucose levels is now in clinical trial. It's called an infrared blood-glucose analyser.

Q **What does it do?**

A The person inserts a finger into a hole in one side of this shoe box-sized device, then the device measures current blood-sugar levels by a process called 'attenuated photo reflection'. In short, measurements are made without drawing blood. In one small trial, scientists found that the analyser's error rate was about the same as the error range of standard finger-prick tests. This high-tech blood-glucose analyser may be on the market soon – but it is likely to be expensive.

Q **Hold on a moment – you mentioned 'error rate' and 'error range'. Are you suggesting that glucose meters aren't accurate?**

A To quote members of the medical profession, a '20 per cent deviation from baseline' is acceptable. Translated, that means blood-glucose readings from meters can be off by as much as 20 per cent and still be valuable.

Q **Isn't that rather a large deviation?**

A At first glance, it seems so. But experts none the less view BGM as more accurate than the urine-sugar test, which was previously the only sugar test people could perform at home – and an imprecise one at that.

Q   **What is the urine-sugar test and why is it imprecise?**

A   The urine-sugar test can detect above-normal blood-sugar levels that occurred a few hours earlier, but it can't give an up-to-the-minute measurement of *blood* sugar, simply because it doesn't test the blood. The level of sugar in the urine represents the blood-sugar levels from some time before. Obviously, blood tests are a far more accurate source of information about blood-sugar levels.

Q   **Going back to glucose meters, what causes a 20 per cent error rate?**

A   Many things. Sometimes it's a matter of improper technique with the lancet or the meter itself. Mishandling the meter, as by dropping it or leaving it in a hot car, can cause it to malfunction. Improper storage of test strips – perhaps exposing them to intense sun or moisture – can lead to a faulty reading. Another part of the blame for misreadings and errors can be put on the quality of instruction that people receive.

Q   **What do you mean? Is there a problem with instruction?**

A   It is clear that many people with diabetes are not taught how to use meters properly – if indeed they are taught at all. It should be the responsibility of doctors, meter manufacturers and nurse diabetes specialists to know all about meters and to make it their business to teach patients with diabetes how to use them. Many monitoring errors result from improper training, misunderstanding of instructional materials and bad habits developed over long periods of unsupervised self-monitoring.

Q   **In the light of these problems, what can people with diabetes do to protect themselves?**

A   The message for all people who practise self-monitoring is clear: be an informed person! Get one-on-one training in meter use, perhaps from two or more people. Ask questions if you get conflicting or inconsistent advice.

Q   **Are there other self-care tests I should know about?**

A   Yes. Besides blood-glucose tests and urine-sugar tests, there is the urine-ketone test (also known as the urine-acetone test).

Q   **What does the urine-ketone test do?**

A   It detects the presence of ketones, acidic toxins, in the blood. Ketones are formed when fat instead of glucose is burned for energy, which happens when there is no insulin in the blood. People with type-I diabetes use the urine-ketone test to check for the life-threatening condition *ketoacidosis*, which leads to diabetic coma.

Q   **Any other tests?**

A   There are several other tests which are discussed later in this chapter – ones that, for the time being, must be done in a doctor's surgery, laboratory or hospital.

Whatever the form, self-testing is only one part of the diabetes self-care routine. Another major element is nutrition – the foods we eat.

NUTRITION

Q   **Why is nutrition so important?**

A   Diabetes is basically a malfunction in the body's ability to use food as energy, so food is an important part of the treatment plan. The kinds of foods a person with diabetes eats, for example, will influence the course of the disease.

Q   **So you're talking about diet here?**

A   Diet or, as it is also called, the eating plan. There are no two ways about it: diet is crucial in the treatment and management of diabetes. That's why people first diagnosed with diabetes are often referred to a dietitian for assistance in analysing their eating habits and forging better eating plans.

Q   **Will a new eating plan call for major changes in the way I eat – restricting certain foods, for instance?**

A   It will be necessary to eat well, following sound nutritional principles. You'll have to make some adjustments, perhaps in how much you eat, perhaps in how often, perhaps in what you eat. Whether or not this is a major change depends upon how you've been eating in the past. While many people with diabetes – especially type-II diabetes – do have to make major dietary changes, what most of them have to do is to learn not to overeat or to make poor food choices.

Q **What are the proper food choices?**

A Evidence from numerous recent studies documents the importance of a high-fibre, high-*complex*-carbohydrate diet in improving glucose metabolism. This is an important and relatively new idea. Before about 1980, doctors had always steered their patients towards a low-carbo hydrate diet.

As you know, food consists of three nutrients: proteins, fats and carbohydrates. Proteins are used to refurbish the body, replacing worn-out body building material. Fats are a semi-permanent form of nutrient storage. You might envision them as an emergency or backup fuel system. But when it comes to keeping the body running (or walking or talking), carbohydrates are the real workhorses of the nutrient family. During digestion, carbohydrates are converted either into glucose or glycogen. Glucose is used for immediate energy. Glycogen is glucose in temporary storage, poised and ready to be retrieved at precisely the moment the body calls for energy.

Q **How much of each – proteins, fats and carbohydrates – is necessary?**

A The latest nutritional guidelines suggest that proteins should account for only 15 to 20 per cent of total calories. An even lower amount is suggested for some people with diabetic nephropathy, a form of kidney disease discussed in Chapter 4. Fats should account for less than 30 per cent and carbohydrates for 55 to 60 per cent. Fibre intake should be about 25 grams a day for women and 40 grams a day for men.

Q **Do these guidelines differ from those that someone who does not have diabetes should follow?**

A No. The high-fibre, high-carbohydrate 'diabetic diet' is the same eating plan now recommended for the general population. It is, in short, a healthy diet. Clearly, the ABCs of good eating apply to everyone, whether they have diabetes or not. For people with families, this is good news: it means a healthy diabetic meal is one that the rest of the family can share.

Q **Must people with type-I diabetes eat different foods than people with type-II?**

A As we said, the basic nutritional principles apply to all, so the foods remain the same. However, the *goals* of diet therapy differ.

People with type-I diabetes follow a simple formula: eating increases blood sugar; exercise and insulin lower blood sugar. For that reason, people with type-I diabetes are very concerned with the timing of their meals. Meals and snacks must be co-ordinated with insulin injections and exercise so that blood sugar always remains within target levels.

People with type-II diabetes must remember that eating increases blood sugar, and that consuming a lot of calories at one time can overwhelm the body's limited ability to use insulin efficiently. This limited ability, or insulin resistance, seems to be triggered or intensified by obesity. As most people with type-II diabetes are overweight, their diet goals centre on reducing food consumption (which reduces insulin demands on the body) and losing weight (which enables what insulin is present to operate more efficiently).

Since food intake affects blood glucose, both groups (people with type-I and type-II diabetes) should take care not to make any major changes in their diet without consulting their doctor.

Q   **Are fats particularly problematic for people with type-II diabetes?**

A   Fats are a problem for most Western people, not just those with diabetes, and the recommendation to reduce fat intake to less than 30 per cent applies to all people. High levels of dietary fat have been shown to increase the risk of cardiovascular disease – primarily through the effects of fats (cholesterol and triglycerides) in the blood.

Fat comes in three forms – saturated, polyunsaturated and monounsaturated – and the recommendation is that people with diabetes eat some of all three, the smallest amount being saturated fat.

Q   **Why is that?**

A   Let's look at where fats are found. Saturated fats come from meat and dairy products, although certain tropical oils (cocoa butter and coconut, palm and palm-kernel oils) are also highly saturated. Polyunsaturated fats come from vegetable oils, including corn, cottonseed, safflower, soya bean and sunflower. Monounsaturated fats are found in olive and canola oils and in avocados. Both polyunsaturated and monounsaturated fats are liquid at room temperature, and they appear to lower cholesterol when they replace saturated fats in the diet.

Q **And lowering cholesterol is a good thing, right?**

A For someone with diabetes, yes. Years ago, diabetes management revolved simply around blood sugar control. Now doctors know that control of fats, or lipid levels, in the blood is also very important. A high cholesterol level is a major risk factor for atherosclerosis, and blood-fat levels tend to be higher in people with diabetes than in people without the disease.

In particular, people with diabetes tend to have higher levels of low-density lipoprotein (LDL), a substance that some call the 'bad cholesterol' because it promotes the deposit of fats on artery and cell walls. In addition, people with diabetes tend to have lower levels of the 'good cholesterol', or high-density lipoprotein (HDL), the substance that draws excess cholesterol out of the body. Triglycerides, the normal form of body fats, are also implicated in heart disease. They occur in the blood as a complex with the protein known as **VLDL**, or very-low-density lipoprotein. These are also higher than normal in people with diabetes.

Q **Are people with diabetes more likely to have high cholesterol levels?**

A For reasons yet unknown, high blood sugar tends to increase cholesterol levels in the blood. Therefore, both type-I and type-II diabetes cause higher cholesterol levels if blood-sugar levels are poorly controlled. For example, extremely high levels of the triglyceride VLDL are commonly found in people experiencing diabetic ketoacidosis.

Q **So lowering blood sugar can lower cholesterol and triglycerides?**

A Yes, it appears that the key to low levels of LDL cholesterol and triglycerides, and high levels of HDL, the good cholesterol, lies in glycaemic control. In a nutshell, that means carefully managing your disease, by using an eating plan, insulin or oral agent, weight loss, exercise or (most likely) some combination of these.

Q **So you're saying I should reduce my cholesterol?**

A If you already have high LDL and triglyceride levels, your risk of heart disease increases with each additional lifestyle risk, such as obesity, inactivity, high blood pressure and smoking. That's because high fat levels, arterial-wall changes, insulin levels, hypertension and obesity are all factors that combine to accelerate atherosclerosis in patients with diabetes. Changing your diet to lower cholesterol can reduce the risk of heart disease. Evidence suggests that for every 1 per cent reduction in blood-cholesterol level, there is a 2 per cent reduction in coronary-artery disease.

Q What if my cholesterol levels aren't really high, merely borderline – is that a problem?

A Total serum-cholesterol levels (the overall amount of cholesterol in the blood) and LDL-cholesterol levels which would be considered borderline for people who do not have diabetes should be a matter of concern for those with diabetes.

Q What does all this mean? What levels should I strive for?

A As usual, specific goals vary from person to person; your doctor can help you to set precise parameters. But to give you an idea of what works for some, here's a list of management goals set by one Metabolic Research Group for its adult patients:

- fasting blood sugar: less than 8.4 mmol/L (150 mg/dl)
- total serum cholesterol: less than 200 mg/dl
- fasting serum triglycerides: less than 250 mg/dl
- LDL cholesterol: less than 130 mg/dl
- HDL cholesterol: over 45 mg/dl in men, over 55 mg/dl in women
- reaching desirable body weight.

Q So how can I lower my cholesterol levels?

A One way is to remove the source of cholesterol in your diet by replacing fat-rich foods with fibre-rich carbohydrates. For a person with diabetes, some very respectable authorities recommend that 55 to 60 per cent of daily calories should be derived from carbohydrates. Your doctor may quote different figures; we've seen the range as low as 40 to 60 and as high as 60 to 70 per cent.

Q But aren't there differences among carbohydrates?

A Yes. Carbohydrates come in two forms: simple and complex.

Q What's a simple carbohydrate?

A It's one that can be quickly converted into glucose. It also causes a swift rise in blood-glucose levels. Simple carbohydrates are often called simple sugars. They include soft drinks, sweets and sugars – table or granulated sugar, brown sugar, treacle, molasses and so forth.

Q I suppose that if I'm concerned about my blood-sugar levels, I should leave sugar out of my diet, altogether?

A Not necessarily. For many people this may come as a surprise: sugar, in moderation, is not taboo. Today's research shows that sugar intake by itself doesn't govern blood-glucose levels. For example, one recent study found that people with type-I diabetes could eat two sugar-laden snacks a day – snacks like brownies and ice-cream – with no effect on blood sugar control! And the American Diabetes Association has given the thumbs up on a teaspoon of sugar, honey, molasses, or other sweetener per food serving. That's twice the amount of sugar once recommended.

In the eyes of many experts, sugar isn't the real culprit behind diabetic complications, so concerns over sugar intake shouldn't overshadow the real dietary concern – excessive food intake and high levels of fat in the diet.

Q **What about artificial sweeteners – are they OK to use?**

A Saccharin and aspartame are valid substitutes for sugar. Unlike sugar, saccharin is calorie-free. Aspartame contains so few calories per serving that no one bothers to count them.

So, as you see, simple carbohydrates, or simple sugars, can have a place in a meal plan, as long as the person with diabetes realizes that sugar offers only empty calories – not exactly helpful if he or she is trying to lose weight. Nor is sugar recommended if the person's diabetes is not well controlled.

Q **OK – so simple carbohydrates are primarily sugars. What are complex carbohydrates?**

A Because their cellular structure is more complex, these carbohydrates take longer to be broken down into glucose and absorbed into the bloodstream. Thus, complex carbohydrates don't increase blood-sugar levels as rapidly as simple carbohydrates. Complex carbohydrates include legumes (like beans and peas), grains (like rice), bread, pasta, fruits and starchy vegetables.

The best complex carbohydrates, according to recent research, are those that contain a lot of fibre.

Q Fibre – that's tough plant material, right?

A Yes. Fibre is the indigestible cellulose material in grains, vegetables and fruits. Fibre can slow the speed at which carbohydrates are absorbed and converted into blood glucose.

The recommendation is that people with diabetes increase their consumption of fibre to 25 grams of fibre for every 1,000 calories. Put another way, that's an average of 40 grams a day for men and 25 grams a day for women. Unfortunately, the average person eats only 11 to 23 grams of fibre daily – meaning that some people need to double or triple their fibre consumption.

Fibre comes in two forms: insoluble and soluble.

Q What's the difference between the two?

A As its name implies, insoluble fibre doesn't dissolve in water. It does absorb water, though, and helps escort foods more quickly through the intestinal system. Foods that contain insoluble fibre include wheat bran, such as that found in whole-grain breads, and certain vegetables and fruits, especially apple skin, raw carrots and beets.

In contrast, soluble fibres dissolve in water, turning into a thick, gelatinous mass that slows down the rate of glucose absorption. Soluble fibres are helpful for people with diabetes because they help to prevent a sharp rise in blood sugar immediately after eating. Foods high in soluble fibre include oat bran, legumes such as lima and kidney beans, corn, apples and oranges.

The general recommendation is that fibre intake should be increased gradually, perhaps by adding one fibre-rich food per week and including a high-fibre food in every meal, to give the body time to adapt and prevent excessive wind, a common side-effect of added fibre.

Q **What does fibre do?**

A As we mentioned, it slows the speed at which carbohydrates are converted into glucose. And when people with diabetes increase fibre-rich foods and decrease fat-laden ones, they can reduce cholesterol and triglyceride levels. Research has shown that people with diabetes who follow a diet of 55 to 60 per cent carbohydrates and 25 grams of fibre per 1,000 calories, can drop their blood cholesterol levels by 15 to 20 per cent and their triglycerides by 40 per cent.

Just as diet lowers blood sugar, so it lowers insulin requirements. People with diabetes may be able to decrease their insulin doses by about 10 per cent; people with type-II may be able to reduce the dose of any oral agent by one-third to one-half. And because high-fibre foods are very filling and low in fat, they can help people to lose weight.

Q **You've been talking about a high-carbohydrate diet. But I've heard that a low-carbohydrate diet is the best one for diabetes. I'm confused. Can you explain?**

A First, we must emphasize that it is complex, high-fibre carbohydrates we have been talking about. Second, it must be acknowledged that the medical profession is rarely unanimous on any issue, and this is no exception.

A few doctors and dietitians still insist that a low-carbohydrate diet is better for some people with type-II diabetes. Some of these doctors argue that a high-carbohydrate meal makes it impossible to attain normal blood-sugar levels for several hours after eating. In contrast, most doctors expect and accept a higher post-prandial, or after-meal, blood-sugar reading.

Q **These conflicting opinions are a little worrying. How do I decide what treatment course to follow?**

A You can't make the decision alone – you must make it in conjunction with your GP, who is your partner in health care. It's always essential for any person with diabetes to delve into issues and discuss them with his or her doctor. The moral is: speak up!

Q **OK, let's say my doctor and I figure out the right balance of protein, fat, carbohydrates and fibre. What's the next step?**

A Decide how much to eat. This is crucial for people with type-I diabetes, because the projected size of their meals determines insulin doses. Once insulin is injected, people with diabetes can't eat more or less than planned without throwing blood sugar off-balance.

Q **What about those of us with type-II diabetes?**

A The amount you need to eat depends upon your age, height, sex and the amount of exercise you get. Your GP or a dietitian can help you map out the appropriate number of calories you need each day. You need to be precise about your calorie needs if you must lose weight or if you are concerned about gaining it – because too much food causes too many pounds.

Q **Is there anything else people with diabetes need to keep in mind?**

A Yes, and that's the frequency of meals. Generally the experts agree that 'small feedings' – three or four small meals a day – are better than one large daily meal.

Doctors recommend that people using insulin should schedule their meals so that they eat something – if only a snack – at peak insulin times. People with type-II diabetes who don't use insulin are encouraged to spread out their caloric consumption into three meals and several snacks, so that they aren't calling on their pancreas to produce large amounts of insulin to cope with one or two large meals. There is another reason for spreading out caloric consumption: people who eat frequent small meals (particularly meals that are high in soluble fibre, which prolongs absorption time) may be less likely to experience the higher levels of cholesterol and triglycerides that accompany diabetes.

Q **Do all complex carbohydrates slow increases in blood glucose?**

A As studies were done on various foods and their effects on blood sugar, researchers discovered that different carbohydrates break down at different rates. The carbohydrates in a potato, for instance, are converted into glucose more quickly than the carbohydrates in rice.

Q **Is there anything that can make meal planning simpler?**

A To help people with diabetes, an idea known as the exchange system has been developed and is widely used.

Q **What's this?**

A Under this system, foods are grouped into six categories: bread and starch, vegetables, fruits, milk, meats, fat. The foods in each category, when eaten in the portions indicated, have the same number of calories and the same nutritional value. For instance, under the bread and starch category, one 'exchange' – one-third of a cup of vegetarian baked beans – has the same number of calories as one 'exchange' – one slice – of raisin bread.

You can see how this makes calorie counting and meal planning less painful – all the calorie-counting footwork has been done. The exchange system helps people accurately co-ordinate their insulin doses with the amount of food they eat. It also helps you to set up a plan to lose weight. As long as people use the specified portions, they can substitute any exchange of one food under a particular heading with an exchange of another food from that same group, knowing that both have the same number of calories and the same nutritional content. You can get tables of exchanges for each of the six groups.

Q **Speaking of nutritional content, what's the official stand on caffeine – is it something people with diabetes must avoid?**

A The amount of caffeine in a couple of cups of coffee or tea or in several soft drinks isn't going to affect diabetes control. For that reason, most doctors say that coffee and tea are fine in the diet. However, as with any kind of food product, moderation is the key. Very large amounts of caffeine (5 to 10 cups of coffee a day) may raise blood sugar. Furthermore, the adverse effects of too much caffeine are often confused with signs of an insulin reaction, or vice versa: anxiety, trembling and irritability.

Q **Can people with diabetes drink alcohol?**

A Most can – in strict moderation, of course. Excessive drinking, however, is likely to wreak havoc with their blood-glucose level, sending it plunging downwards by interfering with the way the liver processes glycogen.

In addition, the diabetic drugs known as oral hypo-glycaemic agents may interact with alcohol, causing facial flushing, severe headaches or dizziness. If that happens, you could ask your doctor to put you on a different oral agent. The new drug might not interact with alcohol, but then again it might – doctors find it impossible to predict who will be affected by which drug. As a result, some people using oral agents find it less aggravating not to drink at all.

If you choose to have an occasional drink (and many people with diabetes do), be aware that alcohol contains calories – and no vitamins. These calories must be accounted for when someone is trying to lose or maintain weight.

Q Do dietary supplements have a role in diabetes care? For instance, do people with diabetes need extra vitamins?

A Many practitioners recommend a daily multivitamin-mineral supplement, in part because they believe that frequent urination (a hallmark of high blood-sugar levels) may discharge needed nutrients, and in part because they worry that a high-fibre, high-carbohydrate diet may lead to vitamin and mineral binding, which is caused when a food prevents a vitamin or mineral from being absorbed during digestion.

In general, the mainstream medical profession is not enthusiastic about large doses of vitamins for anyone, let alone people with diabetes. It has been noted that large doses of vitamin C can lead to unreliable readings of urine-sugar tests – something to keep in mind if you plan to use this type of test.

Q What about fish-oil supplements?

A Eating fish can help prevent coronary-heart disease by lowering cholesterol levels, according to numerous studies. However, while fish-oil supplements may help control cholesterol, studies show that they increase blood-sugar levels. In the long run, the increased blood-sugar levels would erase any benefit of the fish oil on cardiovascular disease.

Today, experts recommend that people with diabetes eat fish, but they advise staying away from fish-oil supplements.

Q **Are there any herbal or homoeopathic approaches to treating diabetes?**

A The plain truth is that diabetes is much too serious a condition to be treated by methods that simply don't stand up to scientific scrutiny. Anyone trying to use homoeopathy to treat diabetes would soon find that this is no substitute for proven methods. Such an attempt would be highly dangerous. All existing herbal remedies of any medical value have already been exploited by pharmacology; the rest are largely useless. And, as recent medical publications have shown, many current herbal remedies, being unstandardized and enormously variable in potency, as well as often being toxic, can be dangerous.

Q **What about vegetarianism? Is it healthy?**

A A carefully planned vegetarian diet can be very healthy. Long-term retrospective studies of vegetarians find that they live longer and healthier lives than their peers eating the typical Western high-protein, high-fat diet. For one thing, vegetarians are less likely to develop heart disease. Legumes (beans and peas), which are staples of vegetarian eating plans, are high in fibre and so are thought to help lower serum-cholesterol levels.

The thing to remember is that there are lots of different foods in the world and lots of opportunities to mix them in creative, satisfying and nutritional combinations. Of course, a 'good' diet or meal plan is not just one that is nutritionally sound – it has to be one that the person with diabetes will eat! In other words, it has to be appetizing to the individual palate. Also, it can – and should – take into account ethnic preferences.

Q **What do you mean by 'ethnic preferences'?**

A Different ethnic groups historically tend to prefer different foods. Since diabetes strikes a disproportionate share of some minority groups, people with diabetes shouldn't hesitate to develop recipes that they find palatable.

Q **What else can you tell me about diet?**

A It's not our goal to be encyclopaedic about nutrition, but we do wish to stress the effect on blood sugar of the foods you choose to eat. There are plenty of sources of more information on fats and carbohydrates; some of them are listed in the Sources of Information chapter which follows this one. If you're interested, search these out. The more information you have about your disease, the wiser you'll become and the better a partner you'll be in your health care.

Q **OK. Let's say I've mastered nutrition. Now can I put my feet up and relax for a while?**

A Not so fast! You'd probably be better off slipping on a pair of walking shoes and heading out for a brisk 20-minute jaunt in the fresh air, because exercise is the third crucial element in the treatment of diabetes.

EXERCISE

Q **What does exercise do?**

A Exercise does many things – it improves one's state of mind, builds muscle tone and speeds the process of losing weight. Most of all for people with diabetes, it lowers blood sugar by making tissues more sensitive to insulin. Twenty minutes of fast walking, for instance, may bring blood glucose down 1 mmol/L (20 mg/dl).

A person with diabetes who is out of shape or just plain new to an exercise regimen may need to check with a GP before launching into an exercise programme. A doctor can give him or her details about the optimum heartbeat rate for someone of the same age, weight and overall physical condition. Since exercise lowers blood sugar, people with type-I diabetes will initially need medical assistance in determining how to adjust food intake and insulin doses on their new exercise plans. In fact, people who are insulin-dependent – or those with type-II diabetes who are on oral agents – need to exercise a few precautions before exercising their limbs.

Q **What precautions are these?**

A They may need to eat before, during or after exercising to compensate for the anticipated drop in blood sugar. Many exercisers who have diabetes carry a small sugary snack in case blood-sugar levels fall too low. If they're insulin-dependent and exercise vigorously, they should inform the people they exercise with, and teach them about the symptoms of hypoglycaemia. Wearing a bracelet or necklace or carrying a wallet card that identifies the exerciser as insulin-dependent is an extra measure of precaution.

Q **What types of exercise are best?**

A Most authorities in the field agree that a three-times-a-week programme of walking, swimming, jogging, bicycling, aerobics, rowing, hiking, cross-country skiing – whatever a person can handle, as long as it gets the heart pumping for 20 to 30 minutes and makes him or her work up a sweat. These exercises, called **aerobic exercises**, build cardiovascular fitness.

Exercise buffs will tell you that it's important to warm up before exercising and to cool down afterwards. Look for flexibility exercises – stretching and bending – to help you loosen up your joints and prepare your muscles for the work ahead. Flexibility exercises reduce the chance of injuring muscles.

Q **You mentioned exercising three times a week. Why does it have to be that often?**

A Frequent exercise is essential because the benefit of exercise on insulin efficiency does not last very long. People who are trying to lose weight might do well to remember that the more often they exercise, the more calories they burn and the more easily they will be able to keep to their diets. Exercising three or more times a week can help people lose weight faster.

Q   **So exercise can be very helpful?**

A   Extremely beneficial for many people with diabetes – and perhaps even crucial for people who have a family history of diabetes but who have not yet developed the disease.

Q   **Why is that?**

A   Research has shown that regular vigorous exercise – the kind that induces a sweat – may protect people against developing diabetes. In a study of 87,253 women from 1980 to 1988, the researchers found that, compared with women who did not exercise, women who exercised vigorously at least once a week lowered by one-third the risk of developing type-II diabetes.

Q   **What kind of vigorous exercise?**

A   Brisk walking, playing tennis, jogging, swimming, hiking, bicycling and the like. *Strenuous* is another word researchers use to describe activities that make you sweat.

Even a simple routine of 'power' walking or swimming several days a week can help. And there's more good news – this study showed that the benefit of exercise held true whether the women were obese, moderately overweight or not overweight, and was beneficial regardless of family history of diabetes.

Q   **What about men?**

A   Recent research has since confirmed the same phenomenon in men. One study, reported in 1992, found that the more frequently the men exercised, the less likely they were to develop type-II diabetes, even in the face of other risk factors, such as smoking, high blood pressure and obesity. Men who worked up a sweat five or more times a week had 42 per cent less risk of developing diabetes than those who exercised less than once a week. Men who worked out two to four times per week reduced the risk by 38 per cent, and those who produced a sweat once a week reduced the risk by 23 per cent.

Q **Can anyone with diabetes exercise?**

A In theory, exercise is good for everyone. It gets the circulation going, lowers blood sugar, increases muscle tone, guards against osteoporosis in women and lowers the risk of heart disease. In people with type-II diabetes, exercise in combination with a well-crafted meal plan can burn off unwanted fat while increasing the body's sensitivity to insulin.

There are some caveats, however. Once someone is relying on insulin (and that includes many people with type-II diabetes as well as most who have type-I), exercise takes on a different dimension. Exercise has to be planned for, and insulin doses adjusted as appropriate. Insulin users should not exercise when they are ill, even if it's something as minor as a cold or flu. Blood-sugar levels are difficult enough to control during illness without adding another variable in the form of exercise. Nor should someone with diabetes exercise on the feet when he or she has a foot injury. Exercise might exacerbate a blister, bruise or cut, resulting in an infection or an ulcer.

Sad to say, too, some people with diabetes can't exercise because their disease has already progressed too far.

Q **In what way?**

A In particular, regular physical activity may not be possible for people who have developed severe diabetic complications. One study that looked at 837 hospitalized people with insulin-treated type-II diabetes found that 69 per cent had at least one complication that precluded vigorous exercise or demanded special precautionary measures if exercise was to be attempted. Granted, these people were hospitalized and so had a more severe form of diabetes than many of their peers. But the lesson is clear : people with diabetes must begin exercise programmes as early in the course of their disease as possible, before it's too late to reap the many benefits.

On the whole, though, exercise is quite amazing, apparently preventing the development of type-II diabetes and helping those who already have the disease to bring their blood sugar into control. Perhaps we might suggest (with tongue only slightly in cheek) that people who are at risk of developing diabetes should run, not walk, to their doctor's surgery to discuss setting up an exercise plan.

Which brings us to a related area of self-care – the proper care of your feet.

FOOT CARE

Q What do you mean by proper foot care?

A For a start, examine your feet every day for even minor problems, such as cuts, corns, bruises and blisters. Left undetected, any one of these seemingly simple problems can lead to a major infection and, if you're very unlucky, gangrene. Diabetic foot disease is the cause of 20 per cent of hospitalizations for people with diabetes, and diabetes-related amputations account for about half of all non-trauma-associated amputations. Fortunately, there are ways to prevent yourself from becoming one of these statistics. Here's how:

- Inspect and wash your feet daily in warm (not hot) water; blot to dry, and do not rub hard between the toes. Use a moisturizing cream (but not between the toes).
- Change shoes twice daily. Wear leather shoes with large toe boxes, such as soft leather jogging shoes.
- Wear clean cotton or wool socks that are the proper size for your feet.
- Don't use hot-water bottles, heating pads or heat lamps near your feet.
- Don't cross your legs when sitting – it reduces circulation in the legs – and don't wear garters.
- Don't cut your toenails – file them so that they are straight across. Slightly round the corners by filing them diagonally.

- Don't use chemical agents to remove corns or calluses, and don't use inserts or pads without checking with your GP.
- Don't wear new shoes for more than an hour at one time until they are broken in, and don't wear shoes without socks.
- Never go barefoot out-of-doors. Sandals and open-toed shoes are invitations to problems.

DENTAL CARE

Q **Do I need to pay special care to my teeth and gums?**

A Yes. Uncontrolled diabetes seems to increase the risk of gum disease – a major cause of tooth loss – and leads to more cavities. Regular dental care (brushing and flossing teeth) and dental checkups are important in people with high blood sugar. Watch for the signs of gum disease, which include bleeding or swollen gums, receding gums and loose teeth, and report them to your dentist immediately.

And talking of the mouth – one thing you should never put in it is a cigarette.

SMOKING

Q **Are you telling me to give up smoking?**

A Yes. But that's something you should really tell yourself. Everyone knows that cigarette smoking increases the risk of heart disease and lung cancer. Smoking definitely poses these risks for people with diabetes — and it has other disadvantages.

Q **Such as?**

A Studies suggest that insulin users who smoke require 15 to 20 per cent more insulin than non-smokers. But the biggest reason to give up smoking is that it increases the risk of diabetes-related complications, such as cardiovascular and kidney disease, by accelerating small-blood-vessel damage. People with diabetes already have higher rates of cardiovascular and kidney complications — why compound the risk?

Q **Is there anything else I should know about diabetes self-care?**

A We'll now take a look at some special situations related to diabetes care. Interestingly enough, these pertain to certain times of life: youth and adolescence, the child-bearing years, and advanced age.

CHILDREN AND DIABETES

Q **Are the treatment goals different for children with diabetes?**

A As with adults, the goal is to keep blood sugar within normal ranges and to prevent the dangerous short-term complications hypoglycaemia and ketoacidosis. Good exercise and eating habits must be part of the treatment plan.

Q **Can children practise self-care?**

A Once they get to be of school age, yes. They can be taught to recognize the symptoms of hypoglycaemia and ketoacidosis, understand the fundamentals of meal planning, and even self-monitor their blood glucose.

Very young children obviously require extra care from parents, and even older children still need supervision to ensure they balance exercise with food intake or don't overindulge in sweets with friends. Teenagers, who are often fiercely independent, may resent having to practise a somewhat rigid meal and medicine routine. They may try to take shortcuts, such as neglecting their BGM. However, the hormonal changes of puberty can make blood-sugar levels less predictable, meaning BGM is required more often rather than less. Parents and doctors may find that they may have to work out some type of compromise with teenagers, trading extra control in one area (BGM, for example) with more flexibility in another (such as the type of food eaten).

There are many excellent sources of diabetes information designed just for young people – both children and teenagers; we list some in the Sources of Information chapter. Use them! And remember, it's never too early to teach self-care – or to practise it.

PREGNANCY AND DIABETES

Q **What about diabetes and pregnancy – what special self-care steps are involved here?**

A Women with diabetes who plan to become pregnant should first get their blood-sugar levels under control, using the strategies we've discussed in this book. Well-managed diabetes reduces the risk of complications during pregnancy, but pregnancy requires extra effort and attention to blood sugar, caloric intake, nutritional balance and exercise. Even with extra care there are potential problems, such as premature birth, an abnormally large baby, difficult birth, or an infant born with respiratory problems, low blood calcium, jaundice or an infection.

The insulin doses and food required to control diabetes change during pregnancy: a woman may need close to three times more insulin by the time she is ready to deliver. The goal, as with all insulin therapy, is to keep blood sugar as near to normal ranges as possible. After the pregnancy, the treatment returns to that used before the pregnancy. Women are encouraged to breastfeed their babies (though this may require additional insulin), as it's good for the health of both mother and child.

Q **What about self-care issues related to gestational diabetes?**

A As you may recall, gestational diabetes is any type of diabetes that first appears during pregnancy. In 95 per cent of cases, it disappears after childbirth.

Gestational-diabetes symptoms are generally mild and not life-threatening to the mother. The condition, however, can pose problems for her infant, including hypoglycaemia and respiratory distress. Most women are able to control gestational diabetes through diet and exercise, although a few go on to use human insulin. Oral agents cannot be used during pregnancy. Self-monitoring of blood glucose is mandatory.

All women with diabetes can expect to undergo additional tests during the course of their pregnancy.

Q **What kinds of tests?**

A These might include foetal tests, such as the **alpha feto-protein** test, to check for possible spinal defects. **Ultrasound** tests check the health and development of the foetus and estimate its weight and size (information that determines whether the baby can be delivered through the vagina or if a caesarean delivery may be required). Other tests may include an electrocardiogram to check heart condition, kidney-function tests, urine-ketone tests and frequent eye examinations to watch for diabetic retinopathy. Women who have moderate to severe retinopathy may need to be examined as often as once a month, because pregnancy speeds the course of this diabetic complication.

On the whole, women with diabetes or gestational diabetes need to get frequent medical attention, with an eye towards controlling blood sugar and pregnancy-related complications.

AGEING AND DIABETES

Q **What about an area of concern further along the line – diabetes and ageing?**

A Blood-glucose levels begin to increase in everyone in their fifties and sixties. And while people may not develop actual diabetes, they may develop impaired glucose tolerance (also called glucose intolerance), or slight elevations in blood sugar. This may be a function of ageing, and it may be related to insulin resistance associated with being overweight. Either way, even slight increases in blood sugar put people at greater risk of cardiovascular problems, meaning that the elderly need to pay special attention to diet and exercise.

Q **Can anything be done about glucose intolerance?**

A Food may play a role in preventing or slowing its onset. In one recently published study, Dutch researchers found that 60 per cent of people aged 64 to 87 who regularly ate fish – usually an ounce a day – were less likely to develop glucose intolerance than people who didn't eat fish.

Q   **What about full-scale diabetes in the elderly. Do the concerns change?**

A   Elderly people with diabetes may have difficulty adhering to their regimen for unique reasons. Vision problems or decreased manual dexterity may make it more difficult to use syringes or glucose meters accurately. Exercise plans become more difficult to maintain. Kidney function also declines with age, which means the elderly face a greater risk of kidney complications. Of course, not all older people with diabetes have these problems – many are robust and healthy. But to make the task of self-care easier on the elderly, some doctors recommend more frequent blood tests, a simple meal plan, and GP visits every 3 months to check for eye and foot problems.

Q   **Speaking of surgery visits, what kind of care should I expect from my doctor?**

A   Choosing a doctor is always a personal matter. You want someone who will listen to your opinions and treat you with respect – in short, someone who will treat you as an equal partner in health care. It's also important to choose a practitioner who will strive to keep you as healthy as possible. And that means a focus on prevention – prevention of diabetes complications.

Q   **What kind of preventive services are recommended?**

A   They include quarterly blood-pressure measurements, twice-yearly foot examinations, annual examinations for diabetic retinopathy by a person sufficiently skilled to find it, regular inspection of gums and teeth (a relatively new recommendation), and certain tests: the **glycosylated haemoglobin**, urine protein, and creatinine clearance tests.

Q   **Could you tell me more about these lab tests?**

A   Yes. One of the newest and most important is the glycosylated haemoglobin.

Q   **Glyco ... what?**

A   The glycosylated haemoglobin test, also called the **haemoglobin A1c test**, measures the number of glucose molecules ('glyco') attached to haemoglobin, the oxygen-carrying substance within the red blood cells. This gives a reading of the average sugar level over the previous 6 to 8 weeks – in contrast to a blood-glucose test, which gives a reading of blood glucose at only one particular moment in time. The higher the average blood sugar, the more of it will get attached to haemoglobin.

The glycosylated haemoglobin test is one of the most important ways of checking overall diabetes control. Performed every 3 months or so, it shows you and your doctor how well your treatment regimen is working by telling where your glucose levels have been, on average, for the last 2 months. The test also shows if the data gathered from BGM are reasonably accurate.

Q   **Are there any other tests?**

A   The following are some of the most common laboratory tests. Certain of these tests should be performed
several times a year; others should be done yearly or
less often, depending upon the severity of your disease:

- Cholesterol test (sometimes called a lipid profile). This
  is actually a series of tests which measure lipids, or
  fatty substances, in the blood. These tests include total
  serum cholesterol, HDL cholesterol and triglycerides.
  They are performed to determine a person's total
  cholesterol, LDL cholesterol and triglyceride levels.
  High levels of these increase the risk of heart disease
  and often are signals of inadequate diabetes control.
- Urinalysis. This screens for urinary-tract infections
  which, if left unchecked, may lead to kidney damage.
- Creatinine clearance. This test measures the filtering
  capacity of the kidneys, and thus is used to monitor
  deterioration of the kidneys. It requires a blood test
  and a '24-hour urine specimen' – that is, all the urine
  a person has produced over a 24-hour period.
- Microalbuminuria. This is a test for traces of protein
  in the urine which reflects early kidney changes; it
  often requires a 24-hour urine collection.

Many other tests may be done depending upon the
severity of your disease. These may include an electrocardiogram, an angiogram or a thyroid function test.
Many of these are geared towards detecting or evaluat-
ing a diabetic complication.

Q **You didn't mention a blood-glucose test. Why is that?**

A At first glance, it might seem that a blood-glucose test should be put at the top of the list of tests. In fact, today's best guidelines insist that BGM should be a personal routine and not just something that is done in a doctor's clinic. If you have read this book carefully you will see that this makes sense. Just be sure to take your notebook with your BGM results to the doctor's, so he or she can see the most recent blood-sugar levels.

Q **It sounds like self-care boils down to my taking responsibility for the treatment of my disease.**

A In many ways, yes. Although you will work closely with your doctor, it's ultimately up to you to make the commitment to control your disease, instead of letting it control you.

SOURCES OF INFORMATION

UK

British Diabetic Association
10 Queen Anne Street
London W1M 0BD
0171–323 1531

British Dietetic Association
7th floor, Elizabeth House
22 Suffolk Street
Queensway
Birmingham B1 1LS
0121–643 5483

British Heart Foundation
102 Gloucester Place
London W1H 4DH
0171–935 0185

The London Diabetes and Lipid Centre
115 Harley Street
London W1
0171–487 4470

National Diabetic Foundation
177A Tennyson Road
London SE25
0181–656 5467

The Nutrition Society
10 Cambridge Court
210 Shepherds Bush Road
London W6 7NL
0171–602 0228

USA

American Diabetes Association, National Center
1660 Duke Street
Alexandria, VA 22314
(800) 232–3472
*Local chapters of this organization will be listed in
your phone book.*

American Dietetic Association
216 W. Jackson Blvd.
Suite 800
Chicago, IL 60606–6995
(312) 899–0040

GLOSSARY

ABSORBENCY:
As used in this context, the term is an indication of how quickly injected **insulin** gets into the bloodstream and thus takes effect

ACETONES:
See **Ketones**

ACUTE:
Of sudden onset and brief duration. Often intense, sharp or severe. *Compare* **Chronic**

ADULT-ONSET DIABETES:
A term formerly used for **type-II diabetes**. An alternative is maturity-onset diabetes

AEROBIC EXERCISE:
Steady activity that causes your heart to beat more vigorously and that may make you work up a sweat

ALDOSE REDUCTASE:
An enzyme thought to play a role in triggering the complications of diabetes

ALDOSE REDUCTASE INHIBITORS:
> A class of drugs that block the action of the enzyme **aldose reductase**

ALGORITHM:
> A simple mathematical chart that can serve as a guide for determining how many units of **insulin** to take and when to take them, depending upon blood-sugar level

ALPHA FETOPROTEIN:
> A test that screens for possible defects of various kinds, especially spina bifida, in an unborn baby

ANGIOGRAM:
> An x-ray of large blood vessels performed after a dye opaque to x-rays has been injected. This outlines the blood column in the artery and reveals any narrowing or blockages

ANTIGENS:
> Substances, such as bacteria, viruses or foreign proteins, capable of stimulating an immune response resulting in the production of antibodies

ARTERY:
> A blood vessel that carries blood away from the heart

ATHEROSCLEROSIS:
> A disease of the arteries in which the inner walls thicken due to deposits of fat, **cholesterol**, degenerate muscle and other substances. Atherosclerosis, by restricting blood flow to organs and limbs, is the immediate and definitive cause of heart attacks, strokes, kidney diseases and gangrene. It is often described, with complete accuracy, as the 'number one killer of the Western world'. Diabetes promotes atherosclerosis

AUTOIMMUNE:

A term used to describe what happens when the body's immune system attacks the body's own tissues

AUTONOMIC NEUROPATHY:

Damage to the nerves that control bodily functions such as the digestive system, urinary tract and cardiovascular system

BACKGROUND RETINOPATHY:

A mild, early form of the most common major complication of diabetes. It is primarily a disease of the small retinal blood vessels in the eye, and features tiny swellings on capillaries (microaneurysms), small blot haemorrhages, yellowish waxy plaque 'hard exudates' and sometimes fluffy white areas ('cotton-wool spots'). Background retinopathy can damage vision if the central macular area of the **retina** is involved with hard exudates. It is, however, generally much less serious than **proliferative retinopathy**

BEEF-DERIVED INSULIN:

Insulin obtained from the pancreases of oxen. This differs from **human insulin** somewhat more than **pork-derived insulin** and is more likely to give rise to antibodies

BETA CELLS:

The cells in the **pancreas** that produce and secrete **insulin** into the bloodstream when blood-sugar levels rise. Beta cells monitor blood sugar and secrete insulin in proportion to the rise

BIGUANIDES:

A class of **oral hypoglycaemic agents** – drugs used to

lower blood-sugar levels in **type-II diabetes**

BLOOD GLUCOSE:

Blood sugar. The body's primary source of energy

BLOOD-GLUCOSE METER:

A device to measure blood-sugar levels. This requires a drop of blood which is usually picked up on a special chemically-prepared strip that is inserted into the meter. Design, however, varies. The blood glucose meter allows frequent checks and provides the individual patient, for the first time, with the means of taking full control over his or her diabetes

BLOOD GLUCOSE MONITORING (BGM):

The technique in which people with diabetes keep track of their day-to-day, and sometimes hour-to-hour, blood-sugar levels by means of a **blood glucose meter**. BGM is now the basis of good diabetes control

BLOOD PRESSURE:

The force of blood against the walls of blood vessels

BLOOD SUGAR:

See **Blood glucose**

BORDERLINE DIABETES:

Another term for **impaired glucose tolerance**

BRITTLE DIABETES:

An uncommon complication of diabetes featuring dramatic swings in blood-glucose levels in spite of attempts at control

BYPASS SURGERY:

A method of re-routing blood around an obstruction in a blood vessel so that the organ or part supplied by the vessel can have its full blood flow restored

CAPILLARIES:

Minute blood vessels that carry blood between the smallest arteries and the smallest veins

CARBOHYDRATE:

One of the three basic sources of energy in food; found in grains, vegetables and fruits

CARDIAC:

Pertaining to the heart

CARDIOVASCULAR:

Pertaining to the heart and blood vessels

CATARACT:

A clouding or opacification of the inner lens of the eye or of its surrounding transparent membrane which obstructs the passage of light. Cataract never causes complete blindness, but, if dense, will cause severe visual disability. Fortunately, the surgical treatment with replacement lens implantation is highly successful so long as the **retina** remains healthy. Cataract tends to occur somewhat earlier in people with diabetes than in those who do not have the disease

CATHETER:

A plastic tube for insertion into blood vessels, the bladder or body cavities, usually to allow injection or withdrawal of fluids

CHLORPROPAMIDE:

An **oral hypoglycaemic agent** used to lower blood-sugar levels in **type-II diabetes**

CHOLESTEROL:

A fat-like substance derived mainly from meat and dairy products

CHRONIC:

Referring to a condition or disease that develops slowly and persists for a long or indefinite period of time. Chronicity has nothing to do with severity but refers only to duration. *Compare* **Acute**

CLOSED-LOOP PUMP:

An implantable **insulin pump**

COMBINATION THERAPY:

Treatment of **type-II diabetes** using a combination of **insulin** and an **oral hypoglycaemic agent**

COMPLEX CARBOHYDRATE:

Carbohydrate made from more complex chains of sugar (polysaccharides) that are digested more slowly and raise blood sugar less rapidly than **simple carbohydrate**. Some complex carbohydrates, such as cellulose and other fibrous substances, cannot be digested by humans because we do not possess the necessary digestive enzymes

CONTINUOUS SUBCUTANEOUS INSULIN INFUSION (CSII):

A form of intensive insulin therapy using an **insulin pump**

CONVENTIONAL THERAPY:

In diabetes, the use of **insulin** to keep blood-sugar levels within certain target ranges; it is less stringent than **tight control**

DAWN PHENOMENON:

A sudden increase in blood sugar that occurs in early morning

DEGREE:

In this context, degree refers to the intensity of effect caused by **insulin**

DIABETES MELLITUS:

A disease resulting from the body's inability to produce or use **insulin**, and featuring high **blood-glucose** (sugar) levels. In uncontrolled diabetes the blood sugar will continue to rise to dangerous levels. Glucose is the principal fuel of the body. Because, in diabetes, it is not available to cells, body tissue, especially muscle, wastes away rapidly and fats are used directly as fuels. This results in the production of acidic byproducts called ketone bodies. If these are allowed to accumulate in the blood, **diabetic coma** will occur, and possibly death

DIABETIC COMA:

A term used for the effect of **ketoacidosis**. Diabetic coma is not caused primarily by high blood-sugar levels, although these, too, are dangerous. Ketoacidotic coma features a shift in the acidity of the blood which, if uncorrected, is incompatible with life

DIALYSIS:

The use of a machine to diffuse out from blood waste products normally eliminated by the kidneys into the urine. Dialysis must be used to preserve life after the kidneys have failed, until a transplant can be done

DIET THERAPY:

The use of a controlled eating plan to lower blood sugar

DURATION:

In this context, the length of time that **insulin** acts effectively after absorption

---

EUGLYCAEMIA:
> Normal levels of blood sugar

FASTING:
> A term normally implying refraining from eating for at least a day, but used in this context to mean not eating for longer than 3 or more hours

FASTING BLOOD SUGAR TEST:
> A measurement of blood-sugar level before the first meal of the day, usually 12 hours after eating

FAT:
> One of the three basic sources of energy in food; found in dairy products, meat, fish, nuts, oils and some vegetables. Fats are a high-calorie source used in the body to store energy. Weight for weight, fats provide more than twice the calories of carbohydrate or protein

FIBRE:
> Indigestible material in grains, vegetables and fruits; see **insoluble fibre** and **soluble fibre**

FRUCTOSE:
> A sugar found in fruits, vegetables and honey

GANGRENE:
> Death of body tissues due to a loss of blood supply. In diabetes, gangrene may result from a general deterioration in the blood-carrying capacity of small blood vessels or from total obstruction to a larger artery when blood clots on top of a plaque of **atherosclerosis**. Gangrene is most common in the extremities, especially the feet. This is one reason why people with diabetes must take particular care of their feet

GESTATIONAL DIABETES:
Diabetes that develops in a woman during pregnancy

GLIBENCLAMIDE:
An **oral hypoglycaemic agent** used to lower blood-sugar levels

GLICLAZIDE:
An **oral hypoglycaemic agent** used to lower blood-sugar levels

GLIPIZIDE:
An **oral hypoglycaemic agent** used to lower blood-sugar levels

GLIQUIDONE:
An **oral hypoglycaemic agent** used to lower blood-sugar levels

GLOMERULI:
Tuft-like structures composed of blood vessels, found in the kidneys, through which waste products in the blood are filtered into the urine. Each kidney has about one million glomeruli

GLUCAGON:
A naturally occurring hormone, produced by the **pancreas**, which increases blood sugar. The action of glucagon is thus seen to be the opposite of that of **insulin**

GLUCOSE:
Sugar; the body's primary energy source

GLYCAEMIA:
Sugar in the blood

GLYCAEMIC:
Pertaining to blood sugar

GLYCAEMIC CONTROL:

Any activity that succeeds in maintaining blood-sugar levels within prescribed or accepted safe limits. Control is effected by **insulin**, which lowers blood sugar, eating, which raises it, reducing food intake, which lowers it, or taking exercise, which lowers it. Control is best confirmed by frequent actual measurements done with a **blood-glucose meter**

GLYCAEMIC INDEX:

Scientific measurement of the effect of different foods on blood-sugar levels

GLYCOGEN:

A storage form of glucose. Glycogen is a polysaccharide – a polymer consisting of many glucose molecules linked together. It is formed in the liver and in the muscles and, when necessary, glucose can rapidly be released for use as a fuel. Glycogen is formed when blood-sugar levels rise, but there is a limit to the amount of glycogen that can be formed, and glycogen synthesis cannot usefully reduce blood-sugar levels

GLYCOSYLATED HAEMOGLOBIN:

A chemical linkage between glucose and the pigment of the red blood cells. This is the basis of a useful test which measures the number of glucose molecules attached to haemoglobin – a means of estimating the *average* blood sugar over the prior 2 months. If a patient's glycosylated haemoglobin figure is high, diabetic control has been poor. Many other body substances can become glycosylated

HAEMOGLOBIN A₁c TEST:

A term sometimes used for the **glycosylated haemoglobin** test

HAEMORRHAGE:

A loss of a large amount of blood from the circulation in a short period of time

HIGH BLOOD PRESSURE:

An increase in blood pressure above normal levels; also called **hypertension**. Abnormally high blood pressure damages arteries, promotes itself, and is probably the major risk factor for stroke. The condition has no symptoms until it reaches a dangerous level, so it must be diagnosed by regular routine testing

HIGH-DENSITY LIPOPROTEINS (HDL):

'Good' **cholesterol**; fat-protein complexes which carry cholesterol from the tissues to the liver and from thence, in the bile, into the intestine. Soluble fibre can bind with bile cholesterol to form a compound which cannot be reabsorbed into the bloodstream and so is lost from the body. Protein is more dense than fats, so high-density lipoproteins are those with a lot of protein and a little fat; low-density lipoproteins have a lot of fat and little protein

HUMAN INSULIN:

Insulin manufactured, usually by genetic engineering techniques, to be chemically identical to the insulin normally produced by the body. Many brands are identified as 'Humulin'

HYPERCHOLESTEROLAEMIA:

Unduly high levels of **cholesterol** in the blood

HYPERGLYCAEMIA:

Unduly high blood-sugar levels

HYPERINSULINAEMIA:

Abnormally high levels of **insulin** in the blood

HYPERLIPIDAEMIA:

Abnormally high levels of fatty substances in the blood

HYPEROSMOLAR COMA:

Dangerous dehydration and loss of consciousness caused by the effects of very high blood-sugar levels. The condition is a possible complication of **type-II diabetes** and should not be confused with **ketoacidosis**

HYPERTENSION:

High blood pressure

HYPERTRIGLYCERIDAEMIA:

High levels of normal body fats (triglycerides) in the blood

HYPOGLYCAEMIA:

Abnormally low blood sugar. Hypoglycaemia is one of the most dangerous short-term complications of diabetes and can occur in both forms. It may be due to too much **insulin** relative to the amount of food eaten; insufficient food intake; or too much exercise relative to food intake

HYPOGLYCAEMIC UNAWARENESS:

The failure of people with low blood-sugar levels to experience or recognize the warning symptoms of **hypoglycaemia**

IATROGENIC:

Caused by medical treatment

IMMUNOSUPPRESSIVE DRUGS:

Drugs used to interfere with some action of the immune system, especially its abnormal attack on some of the body's own tissues

IMMUNOTHERAPY:

A method of treatment which attempts to promote or enhance the function of the immune system in its normal processes of promoting health by defending the body against outside attack

IMPAIRED GLUCOSE TOLERANCE (IGT):

Blood-sugar levels that are higher than normal but not high enough to imply diabetes

IMPLANTABLE PUMP:

A small device inserted under the skin that pumps **insulin** into the body at specified intervals and in doses appropriate to the monitored blood-sugar levels

IMPOTENCE:

Loss of the power of achieving or sustaining a penile erection that allows sexual intercourse. Most cases of impotence are not of organic origin, but men with diabetes may suffer a form that is related to the disease. Diabetic impotence is the most common form of organic impotence

INCREASED RISK OF DIABETES:

A term applied to a person considered to be more likely than average to develop diabetes in the future

INJECTION SITE:

The area of the body where **insulin** is injected

INSOLUBLE FIBRE:

Indigestible material, found in certain grains, vegetables

and fruits, that may absorb water but does not dissolve in it. *Compare* **Soluble fibre**

INSULIN:

A hormone produced by the **beta cells** of the **Islets of Langerhans** in the **pancreas**. *Insula* is Latin for 'an island'. In health, insulin is secreted automatically as a response to a rise in the levels of **glucose** in the blood. Its function is to promote the passage of the fuel glucose through 'ports' in cell membranes into the interior of cells where it is oxidized to provide energy. In the absence of insulin, glucose is prevented from entering cells and accumulates in the blood

INSULIN ALLERGY:

Any adverse reaction to **insulin**. Strictly speaking, true insulin allergy involves the production by the immune system of specific antibodies of the class IgE to beef or pork insulin, and cannot occur with human insulin. The term is, however, sometimes loosely used to refer to any reaction to an insulin injection

INSULIN-DEPENDENT DIABETES:

A term commonly used for **type-I diabetes**. It is, of course, the person, rather than the diabetes, that is dependent on **insulin**

INSULIN PEN:

A convenient device shaped like a pen which is used to inject **insulin** in variable dosages

INSULIN PUMP:

A battery-operated device which pumps **insulin** into the body at specified intervals

INSULIN REACTION:

The effects of low blood sugar (**hypoglycaemia**) caused by too much **insulin**, not enough food or too much exercise

INSULIN RESISTANCE:

A term applied to the case when **insulin** is produced by the body but does not act efficiently

INSULIN SHOCK:

Hypoglycaemic shock caused by an overdose of **insulin**, a decreased intake of food, or too much exercise. It is characterized by trembling, sweating, nervousness, irritability, hunger, hallucination, numbness, pallor and sometimes coma

INTENSIVE THERAPY:

A type of diabetes treatment that strives to maintain blood-sugar levels within certain narrow targets. Also known as **tight control**

INTERMEDIATE-ACTING INSULIN:

Insulin that works more quickly than **long-acting insulin** but not as quickly as **short-acting insulin**

INTRAOCULAR LENS:

An artificial lens implanted in an eye after removal of a **cataract**

ISLETS, OR ISLETS OF LANGERHANS:

Clusters of cells in the **pancreas** that include the **beta cells**, which make **insulin**

JUVENILE DIABETES:

A term once used for **type-I diabetes**

KETOACIDOSIS:

In diabetes, a dangerous condition caused by very high

blood sugars, dehydration and high blood levels of **ketones**

KETONES:

Toxic acids produced by the body when it uses fat instead of glucose for energy. This occurs when, in the absence of **insulin**, cells are deprived of their normal glucose fuel. Coma results if ketones rise above a certain level in the blood. This is called **diabetic coma**

KETONURIA:

Ketones in the urine

KETOSIS:

Ketones in the blood

LACTOSE:

A sugar found in dairy products

LANCET:

A special needle used for pricking the finger to get a drop of blood for use in self-monitoring of blood glucose (BGM)

LATENT DIABETES:

See **Impaired glucose tolerance**

LENTE INSULIN:

Insulin that acts for a longer period than soluble insulin but for a shorter period than long-acting protein zinc insulin (**PZI**)

LIPID:

A fat or fat-like substance. **Cholesterol** and **triglycerides** are lipids

LONG-ACTING INSULIN:

Insulin that takes effect slowly and works for a long period of time

LOW-DENSITY LIPOPROTEIN (LDL):
The complexes of protein and **lipid** that carry **cholesterol** from the liver to the tissues; 'bad' cholesterol, which aids in the deposition of fats on the inside of artery walls in the condition of **atherosclerosis**. See also **High-density lipoproteins**

MACROVASCULAR:
Pertaining to the large blood vessels

MACULA:
The central area of the **retina** responsible for sharp, high-resolution vision

MACULAR OEDEMA:
Swelling of the **macula**, the area near the centre of the **retina**

MARKERS:
In diabetes, genetic signposts on a cell which may indicate the possibility that diabetes will develop

MATURITY-ONSET DIABETES:
An alternative and widely-used term for **type-II diabetes**

MATURITY-ONSET DIABETES OF THE YOUNG:
A paradoxical term sometimes applied to **type-II diabetes** in children and adolescents

METABOLISM:
The totality of the processes of converting food into energy to power the body and to build up body tissues (anabolism); and of the process of breaking down organized cell elements and other body tissues (catabolism)

METFORMIN:
An **oral hypoglycaemic agent** used to lower blood sugar in **type-II diabetes**

MICROANEURYSM:

Small swelling on the smallest blood vessels (capillaries). These can be seen with an ophthalmoscope as tiny dark red or black dots on the **retina**, and are one of the features of **Background retinopathy**

MICROVASCULAR:

Pertaining to the smallest blood vessels

MIXED-SPLIT REGIMEN:

A form of diabetes treatment in which mixtures of intermediate-acting and short-acting **insulin** are given before breakfast and dinner

MONOUNSATURATED FATS:

Fats that may protect against vascular disease by lowering **low-density lipoprotein** (LDL) cholesterol and raising **high-density lipoprotein** (HDL) cholesterol

NEPHROPATHY:

Kidney disease or damage that tends to lead to kidney failure. Nephropathy is one of the major complications of diabetes

NEUROPATHY:

Nerve damage resulting in severe pain or loss of sensation. This is one of the complications of diabetes and may lead to such effects as impotence or partial paralysis of eye movement with double vision

NON-INSULIN-DEPENDENT DIABETES:

A term sometimes used for **type-II diabetes**

NONKETOTIC COMA:

A term sometimes used for **hyperosmolar coma**, the kind that may occur in **type-II diabetes**. *Compare* **Diabetic coma**

NORMOGLYCAEMIA:
> Normal levels of blood sugar

NPH INSULIN:
> A form of **insulin** of intermediate duration of action

ONSET:
> In this context, a term used to refer to the speed with which **insulin** takes effect

OPHTHALMOLOGIST:
> A doctor who specializes in the diseases of the eyes and who performs eye surgery

OPHTHALMOSCOPE:
> A tool used in eye examinations to detect damage to the **retina**

ORAL GLUCOSE-TOLERANCE TEST:
> A series of blood tests used to determine how the body reacts to glucose over a period of several hours

ORAL HYPOGLYCAEMIC AGENT:
> A drug used to lower blood sugar in people with **type-II diabetes**. Also called an oral agent. These drugs act either by forcing the **pancreas** to secrete more **insulin** or by other means

ORAL THERAPY:
> Diabetes treatment with **oral hypoglycaemic agents**

ORTHOSTATIC HYPOTENSION:
> A sudden drop in blood pressure occurring when a person gets up after reclining

PANCREAS:
> The dual-purpose gland, located behind the stomach, which produces **insulin** and **glucagon** as well as digestive enzymes. The former are secreted directly into the

blood while the latter pass along the pancreatic duct to enter the small intestine

PERIPHERAL NEUROPATHY:

Nerve damage in the hands, legs and feet

PHOTOCOAGULATION:

The use of a laser beam to cause controlled damage to the **retina** in the treatment of **proliferative retinopathy** or some cases of **macular oedema**

PLASMA:

Blood from which the cells have been removed

POLYUNSATURATED FATS:

Dietary fats containing unsaturated fatty acids which may reduce **low-density lipoprotein** (LDL) cholesterol

POLYURIA:

Abnormally frequent urination with the production of excessive quantities of urine. Polyuria occurs when blood-sugar levels rise abnormally and the kidneys attempt to dispose of surplus sugar in the urine. The considerable fluid loss causes great thirst. Polyuria and thirst are classic signs of untreated or under-treated diabetes

PORK-DERIVED INSULIN:

Insulin derived from pig pancreas

POSTPRANDIAL:

After a meal

POTENTIAL ABNORMALITY OF GLUCOSE:

A term applied to people who have a close relative with **type-I diabetes**, or people with **islet** cell antibodies

PREVIOUS ABNORMALITY OF GLUCOSE TOLERANCE:

A term applied to people who have experienced

impaired glucose tolerance in the past but have no sign of abnormal glucose metabolism now

PRIMARY FAILURE:

The situation in which an **oral hypoglycaemic agent** fails to lower blood-sugar levels

PROLIFERATIVE RETINOPATHY:

Advanced disease of retinal blood vessels in which new and fragile fronds of small blood vessels extend into the **vitreous humour** of the eye, producing a risk of sight-threatening bleeding. In its advanced stages, proliferative retinopathy leads to the formation of fibrous strands between the **retina** and the **vitreous**. These can contract and pull off the retina. The only hope of restoring vision in advanced proliferative retinopathy is to perform delicate intraocular microsurgery to remove all abnormal tissue

PROTEIN:

The principal structural material of the body from which bones, muscle and connective tissue are made. Also, one of the three basic sources of energy in food. Dietary protein is found in fish, meat, eggs and, in lesser amounts, in grains and legumes

PZI:

Protamine zinc **insulin**; a long-acting insulin

REACTION DENIAL:

A situation in which a person with diabetes does not admit he or she is having a hypoglycaemic attack, usually because blood-glucose levels in the brain have dropped to the point at which the higher brain functions are impaired

RECEPTORS:

Structures on cell membranes and within cells that serve as gateways to the cell, allowing **insulin** and other chemicals to enter

RECEPTOR SITES:

Places on or in cells where receptors are located

RETINA:

The light-sensing surface on the inside of the rear and side walls of the eye

RETINOPATHY:

Any disease of retinal blood vessels. The most common and most important form of retinopathy is that caused by diabetes which has usually been present for several years

SATURATED FAT:

Dietary fat from animal sources which promotes high blood **cholesterol** levels and encourages the development of the serious arterial disease **atherosclerosis**

SECONDARY DIABETES:

Diabetes that occurs as a result of other conditions or circumstances. In many such cases, the diabetes is caused by another disease, medication or chemical. Among the causes of secondary diabetes are pancreatic diseases (especially chronic pancreatitis in alcoholics), hormonal abnormalities (including those that result from the administration of steroids), insulin-receptor disorders, drugs or chemicals and certain genetic syndromes

SECONDARY FAILURE:

A situation in which a previously effective **oral hypoglycaemic agent** suddenly stops working

SEMI-SYNTHETIC:

A term applied to **human insulin** which has been made by chemical modification of **pork-derived insulin**

SHORT-ACTING INSULIN:

Insulin that takes effect quickly

SIMPLE CARBOHYDRATE:

A **carbohydrate** that can be quickly converted to **glucose** during digestion

SIMPLE SUGAR:

A **simple carbohydrate**

SMBG:

An American abbreviation for self-monitoring of blood glucose. Equivalent to the British BGM (**blood-glucose monitoring**)

SOLUBLE FIBRE:

An indigestible material found in certain grains, vegetables and fruits that dissolves in water, turning into a thick, gelatinous mass. *Compare* **Insoluble fibre**

SORBITOL:

A sweetening agent derived from **glucose** and sometimes used in diabetic diets as a substitute for sugar

SPECIES:

In this context, a term used to refer to the source of **insulin**, whether beef-derived, pork-derived or synthetically manufactured

STANDARD THERAPY:

In diabetes, the use of **insulin** to keep blood-sugar levels within certain target ranges. Standard therapy is less stringent than **tight control**

STROKE:

An often devastating event caused either by the blockage of an artery supplying the brain with blood (cerebral thrombosis) or by bleeding into the brain from a ruptured artery or aneurysm (cerebral haemorrhage). The result is a variable degree of interference with brain function, manifested by paralysis, visual field loss, blindness, speech or comprehension defects, or other effects. Cerebral haemorrhage commonly causes death within hours; cerebral thrombosis is usually less severe. Some degree of recovery is common, but serious permanent disability is a frequent sequel of either. Stroke is one of the consequences of **atherosclerosis** and this, in turn, may be a consequence of poorly-controlled diabetes

SUBCUTANEOUS:

Below the skin but above muscle tissue

SUCROSE:

Simple sugar

SULPHONYLUREAS:

A class of **oral hypoglycaemic agents** – drugs used to lower blood-sugar levels in **type-II diabetes**

SYNTHETIC:

In this context, **insulin** produced in the laboratory through a recombinant DNA process (genetic engineering)

TIGHT CONTROL:

A type of diabetes treatment that aims to keep blood-sugar levels within certain narrow limits. Also known as **intensive therapy**

TOLAZAMIDE:

An **oral hypoglycaemic agent** used to lower blood-sugar levels in **type-II diabetes**

TOLBUTAMIDE:

An **oral hypoglycaemic agent** used to lower blood-sugar levels in **type-II diabetes**

TOTAL SERUM CHOLESTEROL:

A measurement of the overall level of **cholesterol** in the blood

TOXAEMIA:

The presence of bacterial or other poisons in the bloodstream

TRIGLYCERIDE:

Normal body fat, each molecule consisting of a 'backbone' of glycerol (glycerine) to which are attached three identical or different fatty acids. The latter may be saturated (contain only single carbon bonds) or unsaturated (contain some double carbon bonds). Triglycerides are liquid oils at body temperature and are contained in thin-walled fat cells under the skin and in the abdomen. They are the principal energy store of the body and can be converted by the liver into **glucose**, when needed. This will not occur so long as the dietary intake exceeds the energy usage. If dietary intake persists to exceed energy usage, obesity is the usual result

TYPE-I DIABETES:

The type of diabetes in which the body has lost the ability to produce **insulin**. Also called insulin-dependent diabetes or juvenile-onset diabetes

TYPE-II DIABETES:

The type of diabetes in which the body can produce some **insulin**, which is either insufficient for the metabolic needs of the body or is, for some reason, ineffective. This type of diabetes usually appears after the age of 40 and is associated with obesity. Also called non-insulin-dependent diabetes or adult-onset diabetes

ULTRALENTE INSULIN:

Long-acting insulin

ULTRASOUND:

A test that uses sound waves to create a picture of organs and structures deep inside the body. It is used, among other things, to check the health and development of a foetus and to estimate its weight, size and delivery date

UNSATURATED FATS:

Fats, mainly of vegetable origin, that are usually liquid at room temperature and, taken in the diet in place of saturated fats, may reduce blood **cholesterol** levels

VASCULAR:

Pertaining to blood vessels

VITRECTOMY:

Surgical removal of the **vitreous humour** from the eye

VITREOUS HAEMORRHAGE:

A **haemorrhage** inside the eye that usually affects vision

VITREOUS HUMOUR:

A clear gel-like material filling the rear part of the eye behind the crystalline lens

VLDL:

Very low-density lipoprotein. A fat/protein complex consisting largely of **triglycerides** linked to a small amount of protein

SELECT BIBLIOGRAPHY

'Audit of diabetes in General Practice', *British Medical Journal* 23 February 1991: 451

'Blood taking for diabetes check', *Lancet* 22/29 December 1990: 1566

'Brittle diabetes', *British Medical Journal* 3 August 1991: 260, 285

'Brittle diabetes course', *British Medical Journal* 25 May 1991: 1240

'Coxsackie virus causing diabetes', *Lancet* 22 July 1995: 221

'Curing diabetes, peptide therapy', *Lancet* 19 March 1994: 684, 704, 706

'Decemberlining nephropathy in diabetes', *New England Journal of Medicine* January 6 1994: 15

'Diabetes, alternative angle', *Science* 30 October 1992: 766

'Diabetes – an autoimmune disease?', *New England Journal of Medicine* 314: 1360

'Diabetes and B-3-adrenergic receptor gene', *New England Journal of Medicine* August 10 1995: 343, 348, 382

'Diabetes and big babies', *British Medical Journal*
10 November 1990: 1070

'Diabetes, blood glucose monitoring neurosis', *British
Medical Journal* 11 February 1989: 362

'Diabetes, blood glucose testing strips', *Practitioner*
22 September 1989: 1208

'Diabetes, cause, autoimmune disease', *Scientific
American* July 1990: 42

'Diabetes, cause, immunology, T cells', *British Medical
Journal* 11 May 1991: 1103

'Diabetes in children under 5', *British Medical Journal*
18 March 1995: 700

'Diabetes and cigarette smoking', *Journal of the American
Medical Association* February 5 1991: 614

'Diabetes control and complications', *British Medical
Journal* 9 October 1993: 881

'Diabetes control cuts complications', *New Scientist*
19 June 1993: 7

'Diabetes control, effect on complications', *Lancet*
22 May 1993: 1306

'Diabetes control reduces complications', *New England
Journal of Medicine* September 30 1993: 977, 1035

'Diabetes, cyclosporin treatment', *Lancet* 19 July 1986:
140

'Diabetes, defective glucose sensor', *New England
Journal of Medicine* March 11 1993: 729

'Diabetes, the diabetic foot', *British Medical Journal*
26 October 1991: 1053

'Diabetes in the elderly, symposium', *Journal of the Royal
Society of Medicine* October 1994: 607–19

'Diabetes, emergency treatment of ketoacidosis', *Lancet* 25 March 1995: 767

'Diabetes, encapsulated cell therapy', *Science & Medicine* July 1995: 16

'Diabetes, encapsulated islet transplant', *Lancet* 16 April 1994: 950

'Diabetes, environmentally induced?', *New England Journal of Medicine* July 30 1992: 348

'Diabetes epidemiology', *British Medical Journal* 18 April 1992: 1021

'Diabetes and the fundus', *Pulse*: 162

'Diabetes in general practice', *British Medical Journal* 6 March 1993: 599, 600, 630

'Diabetes genes', *New England Journal of Medicine* January 7 1993: 56

'Diabetes, genetic basis', *Lancet* 22 August 1992: 455

'Diabetes, glucose tolerance and ambient temperature', *Lancet* 15 October 1994: 1054

'Diabetes and GLUTS', *Lancet* 22 June 1991: 1517; 1991: 1439

'Diabetes, glycated haemoglobin and control', *British Medical Journal* 25 March 1995: 784

'Diabetes, glycated haemoglobin values', *British Medical Journal* 15 October 1994: 983

'Diabetes, human insulin, awareness of hypoglycaemia', *Lancet* 31 August

'Diabetes, immunology in twins', *British Medical Journal* 23 April 1994: 1063

'Diabetes, implanted insulin pump programmed', *British Medical Journal* 17 November 1990: 1143

'Diabetes incidence in children rises', *British Medical Journal* 23 February 1991: 443

'Diabetes, injection pain', *British Medical Journal* 6 July 1991: 26

'Diabetes, insulin resistance', *New England Journal of Medicine* 315: 252

'Diabetes, insulin-secreting implants', *Scientific American* June 1993: 7

'Diabetes and insulin shock treatment', *Lancet* 20 June 1992: 1504

'Diabetes and ischaemic heart disease', *Journal of the American Medical Association* February 5 1991: 627

'Diabetes, long-term complications', *New England Journal of Medicine* June 10 1993: 1676

'Diabetes and maternal deprivation', *British Medical Journal* 20 July 1991: 158

'Diabetes, microvasodilatation in feet', *British Medical Journal* 11 May 1991: 1122

'Diabetes, mitochondrial DNA mutation', *New England Journal of Medicine* April 7 1994: 962

'Diabetes nephropathy', *New England Journal of Medicine* November 11 1993: 1456, 1496

'Diabetes NIDDM, an enigma', *Lancet* 19 May 1990: 1187

'Diabetes, pancreas transplant', *New England Journal of Medicine* July 23 1992: 255

'Diabetes, pancreatic transplant', *Lancet* 13 November 1993: 1193

'Diabetes, pathogenesis, review article', *New England Journal of Medicine* November 24 1994: 1428

'Diabetes practice, the information gap', *Lancet*
    11 January 1992: 97
'Diabetes in pregnancy, British', *Journal of Hospital
    Medicine* December 1990: 386
'Diabetes prevention', *Lancet* 9 May 1992: 1156
'Diabetes, psychological aspects', *British Journal of
    Hospital Medicine* November 1991: 301
'Diabetes, sampling blood glucose', *Lancet* 30 October
    1993: 1068, 1080
'Diabetes, self testing', *British Medical Journal*
    21 September 1991: 696
'Diabetes, skin capillary pressure', *New England Journal of
    Medicine* September 10 1992: 760
'Diabetes, transplants for', *New Scientist* 7 October
    1989: 29
'Diabetes type 1 and pregnancy review', *Lancet* 15 July
    1995: 157
'Diabetes type 2 gene', *Lancet* 28 November 1992:
    1316
'Diabetes, unawareness of hypoglycaemia', *New
    England Journal of Medicine* September 16 1993:
    834, 876
'Diabetic neuropathy diabetes', *New England Journal of
    Medicine* May 7 1992: 1287
'Diabetics who do not have diabetes', *British Medical
    Journal* 7 May 1994: 1225
'Driving and diabetes', *British Medical Journal*
    21 November 1992: 1238, 1265
'Drug, insulin by inhaled aerosol in diabetes', *Journal
    of the American Medical Association* April 28 1993:

2106 'Early nutrition and diabetes', *British Medical Journal* 30 January 1993: 283, 302

'Eating disorders and diabetes', *British Medical Journal* 6 July 1991: 17

'Exercise and diabetes', *Journal of the American Medical Association* July 1 1992: 63

'Genetics of diabetes', *BJHM* 20 April 1994: 387

'Genetics of type 2 diabetes', *British Medical Journal* 17 July 1993: 155

'Glycosylated haemoglobin in diabetes', *New England Journal of Medicine* May 11 1995: 1251, 1293

'Health of the nation and diabetes', *British Medical Journal* 28 September 1991: 769

'How cells absorb glucose in diabetes', *Scientific American* January 1992: 34

'Hypoglycaemia awareness', *Lancet* 13 June 1992: 1432

'Hypoglycaemia awareness', *Lancet* 30 July 1994: 283

'Hypoglycaemia and diabetes control', *Lancet* 5 October 1991: 853

'Hypoglycaemia and intent in law', *Lancet* 27 April 1991

'Impotence in diabetes', *British Medical Journal* 31 July 1993: 275

'Insulin autoimmune syndrome in diabetes, HLA-DR4', *Lancet* 15 February

'Insulin and diabetes complications', *New England Journal of Medicine* July 29 1993: 304

'Insulin factory', *Scientific American* September 1988: 50

'Insulin new drug series', *British Medical Journal* 17 March 1990: 731

'Insulin prophylaxis in diabetes risk', *Lancet* 10 April
    1993: 927

'Insulin resistance in diabetes', *Lancet* 12 December
    1992: 1452

'Insulin resistance in diabetes', *Lancet* 20 August 1994: 521

'Insulin resistance, prevention of diabetes', *New England
    Journal of Medicine* November 3 1994: 1188, 1226

'Islet cell transplant', *Lancet* 2 January 1993: 19

'Linkage of maturity onset diabetes to gene', *Lancet*
    30 May 1992: 1307

'Lucozade glucagon for hypoglycaemia', *British Medical
    Journal* 16 May 1992: 1283

'Microalbuminuria in diabetes', *British Medical Journal*
    31 October 1992: 1051

'Mitochondrial DNA and diabetes', *Lancet* 28 August
    1993: 527

'Monitoring blood glucose easily', *Science* 6 November
    1992: 892

'Needs of elderly diabetics', *British Medical Journal* 1 May
    1993: 1142

'Pancreas islet transplant', *New England Journal of
    Medicine* December 24 1992: 1861

'Pancreas transplants for diabetes', *Lancet* 2 May 1987:
    1015

'Pancreas transplants in diabetes', *Lancet* 1 January
    1993: 27

'Pathogenesis management, type-II diabetes', *Lancet*
    8 January 1994: 91

'Physical activity and type-II diabetes', *Lancet*
    28 September 1991

'Predicting diabetes', *Scientific American* August 1988: 11

'Preventing diabetes', *British Medical Journal* 4 December
    1993: 1435

'Prevention and treatment of complications of diabetes',
    New England Journal of Medicine May 4 1995: 1210

'Self-monitoring blood glucose', *British Medical Journal*
    14 November 1992: 1171, 1194

'Self-vaccination halts diabetes', *New Scientist* 10 August
    1991: 19

'Shared care in diabetes', *British Medical Journal*
    21 January 1995: 142

'Smoking and diabetes', *British Medical Journal* 4 March
    1995: 555, 560

'Transplant for diabetes', *Lancet* 9 June 1990: 1371

'Treating diabetes with transplanted cells', *Scientific
    American* July 1995: 40

'Type 2 maturity onset diabetes treatment', *New
    England Journal of Medicine* November 12 1992:
    1434, 1453

INDEX